SIMPLE. NATURAL. HEALING.

SIMPLE.
NATURAL.
HEALING.

A Commonsense Approach to
TOTAL HEALTH TRANSFORMATION

Donna LaBar

New York

SIMPLE. NATURAL. HEALING.
A Commonsense Approach to
TOTAL HEALTH TRANSFORMATION

Published in New York, New York, by Morgan James Publishing. Morgan James and The Entrepreneurial Publisher are trademarks of Morgan James, LLC. www.MorganJamesPublishing.com

The Morgan James Speakers Group can bring authors to your live event. For more information or to book an event visit The Morgan James Speakers Group at www.TheMorganJamesSpeakersGroup.com.

Shelfie

A **free** eBook edition is available
with the purchase of this print book.

CLEARLY PRINT YOUR NAME ABOVE IN UPPER CASE

Instructions to claim your free eBook edition:
1. Download the Shelfie app for Android or iOS
2. Write your name in **UPPER CASE** above
3. Use the Shelfie app to submit a photo
4. Download your eBook to any device

ISBN 978-1-61448-543-8 paperback
ISBN 978-1-61448-544-5 eBook
ISBN 978-1-61448-545-2 audio
ISBN 978-1-63047-877-3 hardcover
Library of Congress Control Number:
2015919184

Cover Design by:
Rachel Lopez
www.r2cdesign.com

Interior Design by:
Bonnie Bushman
The Whole Caboodle Graphic Design

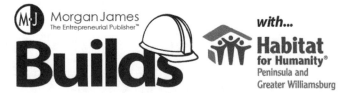

In an effort to support local communities, raise awareness and funds, Morgan James Publishing donates a percentage of all book sales for the life of each book to Habitat for Humanity Peninsula and Greater Williamsburg.

Get involved today! Visit
www.MorganJamesBuilds.com

DEDICATION

This book is written for my daughter and fearless warrior, Monica LaBar Hughes, who taught me to face my fear and do it anyway.

For my dear friend Catherine Garbus and her wonderful father, Allen Garbus, for opening the door and sharing their passion and journey of discovery of the body's amazing ability to heal.

For my dad, Bob Cook, for encouraging my inquisitive mind and teaching me to problem solve with resourcefulness and common sense.

For anyone who is struggling to maintain his health or to share in the struggle of a loved one's serious illness.

This writing is offered to give hope, nutritional healing guidance, and support to guide you back to wellness.

CONTENTS

FOREWORD

It is a pleasure to write the foreword for this book. Donna LaBar has provided all of us with an understanding of how you can help yourself and make a difference in your own health. After many years of knowing there are answers for healthy healing, Donna has given us the information to work with on a daily basis. We are all born with an inherent ability to heal, and when the body receives what it needs, miracles happen and healing begins.

Donna has such passion and drive to help people know there are many nutritional pathways for lifelong health and disease prevention. Her journey was tested when her own daughter needed all her expertise and support. Learning from someone who has gone through a personal journey that ended with the best outcome for health and healing, you will get many benefits when you use this book as a reference.

Donna and I share many similarities in that we've both witnessed how the body responds to proper nutrition and lifestyle changes. She began to study nutrition as medicine to overcome serious health issues in her family and for friends, and over the years, her explanation of healing has helped many people regain their health. What started as curiosity about health has become a mission to share with her readers the importance of knowing and committing to lifestyle changes. She does not simply tell you why it is crucial to get the right information, but she also provides you with an intelligent game plan for success with simple recipes and pantry changes. She is the active partner on your journey to improvement.

The topics discussed throughout the book are for your understanding, to study and become familiar with so that you are ahead of your own health care. The latest statistic is that one in three females and one in two males will experience a cancer diagnosis. With the information presented throughout this book, you can begin today to have the odds in your favor. Keeping yourself healthy requires diligent work on your part and learning all you can do for prevention because well-being is definitely available when you have tools that you choose to use. You will see that miracles don't just happen, but they can be expected when using the information guide provided in this book. Healing is a journey, achieved one step at a time.

I encourage you to grow with the book and use every word to increase your understanding of how to help yourself to win the best outcome for your own journey. With the information at hand and the enrichment you receive from knowing, you can create your own healthy healing journey and duplicate it with friends and family. I am excited for you now that you know what is in your hands.

I honor Donna LaBar, who took the time to present us all with this gift of knowing.

Denise Abda

www.deniseabda.com

ACKNOWLEDGMENTS

This book was a labor of love that took over three years to write, and I have many to thank.

Sybilla Lenz of Positive Living by Design, my soul expansion friend, thank you for taking me to Tony Robbins's event, "Unleash the Power Within," in NYC and then to hear Brendon Burchard in California the same year; this book was born from those adventures!

Erica Glessing of Happy Publishing, San Jose, California, thank you for discovering the best part of me and insisting I write a book about it. Your excitement about my message and help with my book proposal led the way to this writing.

Rick Frishman, thank you for personally giving me encouragement to learn more about being a better author.

Emelyn Smith Fuhrman, thank you for the love and patience you offered during my very first round of edits.

Bob Lizza, thank you for technical support, love and lightheartedness, and for keeping me from taking myself too seriously.

Angie Kiesling of SplitSeed, thank you for guiding me through to the finished manuscript.

Morgan James Publishing, thank you for your expert guidance, not only in writing this book but also in teaching me the greater importance of spreading my message.

For my relatives, friends, and clients who have patiently waited for "the book," thank you for your ongoing encouragement and support.

Chapter 1

TURNING HEALTH AROUND

The new normal of health terrifies me. Acid reflux, hemorrhoids, hiatal hernia, gas, bloating, chronic headaches, rashes, chronic anxiety, insomnia, unexplained and unhealthy weight gain, fluid retention, high cholesterol, high blood pressure . . . No one is scared; it's just *normal* stuff, and the doctors have medicine for all of it. So why am I worried when no one else seems to be?

I'm an American living in a rural community within driving distance of a few major metropolitan areas. I see it in the country; I see it in the city. Our population, for the most part, has become convinced that this is just normal stuff. I've heard it all: "This stuff kills me, but I love it and eat it anyway"; "Saved by the purple pill!"; or "I guess I'm just getting old." And this is from people who are not even fifty! Even worse, I hear some resign themselves to an unhealthy fate: "My kids are heavy like my family"; "My whole family is overweight and has a history of diabetes; it runs in our genes"; or "Heart attacks and strokes run in my family." I could go on, but I'm truly writing this from a place of love and wellness, so I'll get to the point.

1

All of this is *not* normal. These are the warning signs of more hardships and illnesses to come. Eventually disease will come, which may have been avoided if the early warning signs had been taken seriously. Instead, the common response is relief that there's a pill out there that provides temporary help, thus giving a false premise that this is just normal stuff—just take the pill.

The following statistics from a 2014 report by the American Diabetes Association are a perfect example of a disease that is commonly treated in the early stages with a pill.

Overall numbers: diabetes and pre-diabetes
Prevalence: In 2012, 29.1 million Americans, or 9.3 percent of the population, had diabetes.

In 2010, the figures were 25.8 million and 8.3 percent.

Prevalence in Seniors: The percentage of Americans age sixty-five and older with diabetes remains high, at 25.9 percent, or 11.8 million seniors (diagnosed and undiagnosed).

New Cases: The incidence of diabetes in 2012 was 1.7 million new diagnoses per year.

Pre-diabetes: In 2012, 86 million Americans age twenty and older had pre-diabetes; this is up from 79 million in 2010.

(Source: http://www.diabetes.org/diabetes-basics/statistics/, accessed February 18, 2016)

While this data is crazy and so frightening, I don't blame this on the doctors or the population. Doctors want to help people feel better and enjoy a better quality of life. People want to enjoy their life, work, family, and friends. It's that simple. But the world is changing. These statistics have created such a burden on society that change is a must. We can no longer afford such high medical costs, and there are not enough doctors, nurses, programs, and facilities to handle this staggering demand on the health-care system.

It's not the fault of the government workers, employers, doctors, testing labs, or the pharmaceutical industry. It has just come to this. Every individual in those statistics is part of the problem. The change must come from everyone doing his or her part to improve health; this is something we do have control over.

Encouragingly, some individuals are taking the initiative to find solutions for their health issues outside of traditional medicine. This realization and the free access to research any topic via the Internet have allowed a whole new avenue of exploration for individuals who want to take control of and responsibility for their own health and wellness. There is definitely a movement to be more proactive with health, to have a better understanding of what causes illness, and to have knowledge of the alternative lifestyles, programs, treatments, and therapies that are available. Recently I held a one-day, free educational natural-health clinic in our small county with a population of less than thirty thousand, and over one thousand people came out to participate.

I did some quick research to see how many searches there are monthly on the Internet search engine Google for a few topics that plague individuals every day. The results are shocking, but nonetheless, they prove my point: There is a movement in full swing to get more information to resolve common health issues at home. Some of the top concerns are listed below.

Average number of monthly searches
- Diabetes: 1,000,000
- Cancer: 550,000
- Arthritis: 450,000
- Weight Loss: 210,000
- Pain: 201,000
- Sleep: 201,000
- Stress: 368,000
- Anxiety: 450,000

- Constipation: 301,000
- Diarrhea: 550,000
  (Source: https://adwords.google.com/KeywordPlanner/Home, accessed February 9, 2016.)

We have been treating the symptom and accepting illness instead of recognizing the symptom's true purpose: the body is warning us that things are not working properly. The warnings mean, "Change what you are doing!" The body is failing because its basic system is not being supported. It cannot run the way it was designed to run without the basic, necessary components. If a combustion engine was filled with water instead of gasoline, it would go nowhere, and it would have diagnostic problems, for sure. The same applies to us. When the body isn't given the right support, it doesn't have any energy; it starts having performance and quality issues, and then it breaks down.

The human body is designed so incredibly, with such an amazing capacity to do things that science cannot duplicate. Just one of the magical things the body does is to repair and heal itself. It's imperative, therefore, to have the right tools, whether trying to lose weight, get over a nagging illness, or support the body while going through a series of medical treatments, surgeries, or therapies. Once these basics of natural health maintenance and recovery are spelled out, made clear, and feel simple to implement, healing comes naturally—the ultimate reward.

Chapter 2

LIVING THROUGH
A DIAGNOSIS

R ealizing you're still alive after hearing the worst news is a step toward healing. My daughter, Monica, and I lay in each other's arms, frozen in time on her hospital bed, both sobbing with the harsh reality of the news we'd just received. The doctor had politely left us alone to compose ourselves before a child-life social worker came in.

Monica, my only child, had always been a busy girl: a member of the cross country team, a good student, and an entertainer amongst her friends. In the fall of 1998, when she began seventh grade, everything was fine. By the end of September, she was complaining of hip pain. Her cross country coach said Monica should not be in that much pain in the early stages of training because she had been running all summer with the team. The coach thought I should take her to a sports podiatrist to see if she needed orthotics for her shoes. I took her suggestion and made an appointment, which was two weeks out. By the time the appointment came, Monica was sick with flu-like symptoms. She ended up in the emergency room on a weekend in early October with a very high fever.

The hospital took blood work and sent it to our family doctor. We were sent home with instructions for rest and fluids.

The following Monday, our doctor, a kind, soft-spoken woman named Dr. Stone, called with the news that the blood work had a high sedimentation rate. The sedimentation-rate (sed rate) blood test measures how quickly red blood cells (erythrocytes) settle in a test tube in one hour. The more red cells that fall to the bottom of the test tube in one hour, the higher the sedimentation rate. She suggested we get Monica to a larger medical facility immediately. She set up an appointment for us with an infectious-disease doctor.

The medical center was three hours from our home. When we arrived, a gentle, older doctor saw us. He told us that he would run a series of tests; he thought it was a virus and told us that a lot of times patients get viruses that are never identified. He also sent us home with instructions for rest and fluids, with a follow-up appointment scheduled for the next month.

Monica was still very sick by the next appointment. She was weak and had lost a lot of weight. The doctor still felt the same: it was a stubborn virus, and we had to wait it out. Three weeks later, in late November, she was admitted to the children's hospital, weaker than ever. We were still looking for an answer, but when it came, we were shocked. We hadn't considered cancer. Acute myeloid leukemia was the diagnosis.

Monica was extremely ill at this point, and the doctor did not waste any time. They gave us the bad news and our choices. There was no protocol for AML in a child at that time; patients with this kind of leukemia were usually in their seventies or eighties.

A children's cancer study was a possibility, and that would randomize her to a protocol, which would follow her case and document everything for research. It was either this chemotherapy protocol or the other choice: no treatment. In their opinion, she had about two weeks to live without treatment.

We chose the cancer study and waited for the child-life social worker to tell us what to expect in the days ahead. The protocol was three large doses of chemotherapy, each with long recovery periods in between, mostly all in-hospital.

I tried to think of something soothing to say to Monica, who was normally a very witty and silly kid. All I could think to say was, "I don't feel like you are going to die, honey. I just don't feel it." Monica said she didn't feel like she would die either and wanted to do everything possible to get well. I remembered the old saying that you eat an elephant one bite at a time. We had to look at cancer like it was an elephant. We didn't want to tackle the elephant; we thought it was impossible. Some days we would be able to eat a lot, other days only a little, and some days we would just rest. Eventually, we would eat the whole elephant.

I promised her and myself in that moment that I would learn everything I could about this disease, that I would stay by her side, and that I would apply everything I knew about healing in order to help her. I would work with the medical staff, ask every question, and leave no stone unturned.

Monica's treatments started the next day. I spoke to her oncologist, a salty, old, sea-captain-looking man with kind eyes and a quick wit, and explained that I believed in nutritional healing and wanted to work the things I knew into our treatment plan. Over the years, my fascination with the body's ability to heal had led me to study all kinds of nutritional healing topics. Eating an alkaline diet while trying to give the body the best chemistry to recover from illness and enjoy optimum health was something that I had read in many different sources. I also was well informed about vitamins, nutrients, and antioxidants and wanted to have the ability to use everything I could to give Monica the best chance for recovery. Her doctor agreed that it wouldn't be a problem introducing the alkaline foods and supplements after the chemotherapy had spent a week in her system.

So that was our edge. I had a built-in cot in Monica's hospital room where I slept, and it had storage drawers underneath. I stored lemons, peppers, cucumbers, and other fresh fruits and vegetables in the drawers, along with vitamin supplements. I began to work on getting Monica's body back to an alkaline state as soon as I was given the green light after each round of chemotherapy. She had such a small window of being able to eat, so I had to be prepared. Her appetite would decline and then she would get mouth sores, a side effect of her chemotherapy, and she would then ride through the rest of her recovery cycle with very little food.

During the times she couldn't eat, we tried everything else: stress-reduction techniques, pressure-point therapy, massage therapy, guided meditations, visualization meditations, Reiki, and anything and everything that was suggested by other families with a cancer patient or by our own friends and family.

The reality of what the body goes through and has the ability to come back from is unimaginable. Monica had fifty-seven blood transfusions and thirty-four platelet transfusions and had incredible allergic reactions, not only to the transfusions but also to most of the drugs she took. She had rashes on top of rashes. The interesting thing for me was her constant blood work. It gave me the opportunity to see her cells on a daily basis in all stages of decline and recovery. This information gave me a tremendous window inside her body to see how what she ate impacted her cell recovery.

This was an immensely difficult period in our lives, but I learned so much about healing, integrating alternative approaches with standard medical care, and the powerful ability of the body to recover. It was nothing short of amazing.

Monica was in the hospital, predominantly inpatient, for over nine months, with many close calls in the intensive care unit as a result of pneumonia and low potassium. Her potassium became so low from her medications that her heart would not beat properly. During those frightening times, we still, when possible, kept up with our own plan of alkalinity and supplements, and she would eventually rally and start recovering again.

Monica finished with the protocol in August of 1999 and was officially in remission. She had been in a wheelchair for so long that she needed some physical therapy to get up to speed in order to start school. Once she returned, she got back to her life, back to her friends and her studies, but we had both changed. A new awareness and keen understanding about the suffering that happens with a cancer diagnosis brought us both to a place of being able to and wanting to reach out to others who were going through what we had experienced.

An interesting sidebar: Monica went back for regular checkups with her oncology team at the medical center for ten years; it was part of our initial agreement to be in the cancer study. At one follow-up appointment, I asked her doctor if they still used the protocol that she was randomized to. He said they didn't use any of the protocols from the study as they had proven to be ineffective. If a child came in now with AML, they went right into bone-marrow transplant. Five years after that conversation, Monica's oncologist contacted her to see if she would continue to be studied as they were going to revisit some parts of her protocol in their quest for better recovery rates.

Funny how the twists and turns of life end up preparing you for more twists and turns of life. In 1976, I had a job as a legal secretary in a local law office, and a new, young attorney, fresh out of law school, came to work there. Her name was Catherine, and she was from the West Chester area of Pennsylvania. She and I became good friends. In long conversations, we shared stories about our pasts and how we were raised. She introduced me to vitamins and nutrients, a topic I had never considered. Back then, I was curious about them and started taking vitamin B for energy and vitamin C for my immune system. I experienced some improvement, so I continued to read about vitamins and nutrition out of personal interest.

A few years after we met, Catherine's father, Allen, at sixty years of age, was diagnosed with stomach cancer. He was a chemical engineer by profession and, therefore, took a scientific and investigative approach to his illness. He learned that his stomach would have to be removed in order for him to have a chance to live, and his doctors prescribed chemotherapy but didn't give him much hope. Allen did not believe in the logic behind chemotherapy, so he refused it. Allen approached his diagnosis like a scientist. He knew he would have to adjust to living without a stomach, which meant eating enzymes with his food for the rest of his life in order to digest it. This traditional meat-and-potatoes guy had to learn how his body worked to digest his food and had to research how to eliminate the chance of ever having cancer again.

As he was learning, I stayed in touch and learned with him. I was so intrigued. I couldn't get enough information. He and I forged a relationship over the years; through visits, phone calls, and e-mail, we bonded over nutrition and nutritional healing. Because he was a chemist, Allen studied his body at the cellular level. His findings were too complicated for me, so I had to sort them out for my own understanding.

Allen would come up with recipes to heal illnesses he never had. One of them was a good recipe for healing arthritis. We weren't interested in making it, just helping people heal, so I went out in search of a product on the market similar to his recipe. I found a similar product through Life Extension and still have friends who swear by it today. We did this with many illnesses, just to help one of his friends or someone I knew suffering with an illness. This went on for decades; we enjoyed such a beautiful friendship and learned so much together.

Allen died in April 2008 at the age of ninety-three. I loved his stories, his reasoning, and his exceptional wisdom about how the body works. My last visit with him in West Chester was in the late summer of 2007, when he wanted me to come to visit him to review the properties of octacosanol and policosanol to see if either had an advantage to give him more energy. After three hours of clicking through files on his computer and exhausting the topic, I told him to just eat some beets with the green tops from his lovely garden and let it go. He laughed and resolved to do just that.

I grew up in rural northern Pennsylvania. Almost everyone lived or worked on a farm. I was raised in a typical 1950s household: my mom was a stay-at-home housewife, and my dad worked hard as a mechanic to feed his family. I was the eldest of four children, and we had a meat-

and-starch diet with little fresh or raw fruits and vegetables other than during the garden season. We drank Kool-Aid-type drinks and had ice cream and candy for snacks. I remember my mom being excited about hamburger and tuna helper being introduced to the market. It seemed so slick and easy!

Like many adults in the 1950s and 1960s, my parents also smoked cigarettes. In the long run, this has had a very negative impact on my family's health. My mother died in her sleep at the age of fifty from a heart attack, and my father suffered a heart attack and buildup in his carotid arteries in his early sixties and was treated for years for high blood pressure, high cholesterol, and acid reflux. My siblings have also had similar symptoms and, in addition, have also been diagnosed with pre-diabetes and diabetes.

The information I learned and practiced with Allen opened my mind to a whole new world of thinking about food and health, and I am grateful to have good health and to have avoided the need of medications to maintain my well-being.

In my area, a lot of people have low wages and struggle to make ends meet. They also still eat the way my family did back in the 1950s and 1960s, but with the added complication of today's packaged goods and fast foods. Some people think they eat better than average, yet they still see a lot of health issues. They are suffering from so many different ailments, like cancer, diabetes, MS, lupus, and autoimmune disease.

Witnessing people suffering with health issues and hearing the stories of what they go through to find avenues to get well spur me onward to continue what Allen taught me years ago. Getting the word out about what the body really needs to heal and which foods, products, methods, and therapies are available to make the biggest difference in the quickest amount of time is what really brings about change.

There's no complicated diet, magic drink, or crazy stuff to do. There is only the knowledge of how the body functions, produces energy, and repairs itself. The only prescription is understanding the body and what it needs to make its processes all happen optimally.

Chapter 3

THE BIG PICTURE OF HEALTH RESTORATION

All bodies function basically the same. Yes, we all differ in many respects, but the body as a matter of operation, for the majority, runs primarily the same. Eating food provides energy; sleeping provides rest, healing, and rejuvenation; and elimination provides an avenue to detoxify and remove waste from the system. If the body is still functioning without disease, but not optimally, addressing each of these areas at the same time will have a dramatic, noticeable improvement on one's overall health.

If the body is experiencing disease of some sort, then extra support must be given to certain functions to stop the decline of health, stabilize the system, and then move toward recovery. I call this slowing down the train of declining health and then slowly getting it into reverse and moving in the opposite direction toward wellness. Learning new approaches, having hope, keeping the mind focused on wellness, and giving the body the benefit of a healing environment provide the highest probability of restoring health.

There is a basic framework that must be addressed for everyone to enjoy better health, but more must be done, in addition to the basics, to recover if the body has reached a place of disease. The chapters ahead provide the building blocks for the maintenance and recovery of health. Extra information has been provided for diabetes, cancer, autoimmune diseases, and weight loss as they are major health topics that are making a detrimental impact on society.

There are areas of health, such as pH balance and proper acid-alkaline balance, that are crucial but sound like complicated science when mentioned. My task is to sort all this out. I will suggest ways to easily find out if the body is more alkaline or acidic and then provide simple explanations, a chart of alkaline foods, and uncomplicated approaches to reach and maintain the optimal balance. You will then have the greatest noticeable experience toward healing.

There are actually four areas I believe to be of highest importance when it comes to food consumption. Once the four areas of food consumption are addressed, the platform for the greatest healing potential will be in full swing. These areas are (1) alkalinity/acidity, or pH balance, (2) enzymes, (3) digestion and absorption, and (4) anti-inflammatory food choices. I believe that as long as the body can still ingest, there is potential to heal. The areas outside food consumption that equally need to be addressed and have a fresh, new approach are elimination, sleeping, and the way we process thoughts and stress. Each has an impact on health and the recovery to wellness; thus, no stone can be left unturned.

Exploring all the important aspects of natural healing and finding what works best for your current health scenario is key. It doesn't sound like much, but just some clear explanations of these four areas can make a world of difference in health. While it may seem overwhelming, none of this information is very complicated or rocket science. It just needs to be sorted out and delivered in a clear and concise way. Many health conditions can be reexamined in a new light. The approaches I explain present a logical pathway to improved health and a window of opportunity to avoid or overcome illness and disease.

The biggest obstacles are breaking old habits, getting support from family and friends, and having the energy and courage to stay the course. So many try something new for a day or a week and then give up. It takes a while to turn health or an illness around. But with the right information and coaching and with the encouragement gained by witnessing quick improvement, these approaches will easily become a lifestyle.

Chapter 4
THE POWER OF ALKALINITY

Envision the digestion process of the typical American diet as a busy traffic cop with a sad face standing at the processing center. He is frantically trying to figure out what the heck just arrived in the stomach, shouting orders to hose it down with large amounts of acid, demanding the pancreas to send massive quantities of enzymes and hormones. In the chaos, many chunks of food go through unchecked because of the overload on the system, later to be diagnosed as leaky gut syndrome. Then everything slows down as the poor traffic cop witnesses what he dreaded but couldn't control: acid reflux, bloating, cramps, gas, low energy, fatigue, and constipation or diarrhea.

Now imagine a different day, with the same traffic cop but a totally new story: the ease of introducing a pH-balanced diet with enzymes has been discovered. A balance of alkaline and acidic food arrives in the form of food balanced with nutrients, minerals, healthy fats, and proteins. The smiling traffic cop welcomes the oncoming parade of food and personally escorts it through, calmly and efficiently. The easy sorting and processing will optimize the energy and nutrients available to the body. Instantly a new platform has been provided for supported repair and healing to a complex biochemical system.

Many know that the body maintains an internal temperature of 98.6 degrees Fahrenheit, and if that temperature varies by five or six degrees in either direction, the body will react with illness and possibly death. The body has the same internal mechanism for regulating the pH balance of the blood. Many chemical responses happen in the body throughout the day to maintain a slightly alkaline balance of 7.365. When the pH balance drops toward acidic, or under seven in the blood, illness, disease, and possibly death can occur.

When I first studied the body's natural healing process, I saw in most of the readings that I should test my body's pH balance with litmus paper. This was decades ago. There was no Internet, and my local pharmacy didn't know what I was talking about. While I wasn't able to test, I was always curious about my body's pH level. Now you can easily get test strips at the health food store or online. Typically, the strips test the alkalinity of the saliva or the urine. The urine test is actually more accurate because it is testing post digestion. It is simple and painless. The test strips are simply dipped in the urine stream then checked for the alkalinity level by color, with a color chart provided with the product.

If the urine tests acidic, it is an indication that the diet is not supporting the intricate system in the body to supply oxygen, vitamins, and nutrients to the cells through digestion. If this goes on for a long period of time, the body will slowly break down, with warning signs along the way, to a point of dysfunction and illness or disease. I have learned that it's best to consistently test first thing in the morning because the alkalinity of the urine changes throughout the day, depending on food intake, stress, sleep, and other factors. In the morning, the body is fresh from a long period of rest and fasting, giving a consistent status for reading. A consistent good reading assures that the diet is supporting the normal blood pH balance.

Alkalinity in the body happens as a result of the mineral content in our food. The primary minerals that have an alkalizing effect are calcium, iron, magnesium, manganese, and potassium. In order to support the body to maintain the alkaline state, we need to eat foods rich in primary minerals. These minerals are all very important for pH balance, and all of them have different health benefits.

Calcium is a mineral found in the body and in food. Most calcium in the body is stored in our bones and teeth, but it has many important functions in addition to building strong bones and teeth. It also regulates muscle contraction, nerve conduction, and cell-membrane function; regulates enzyme activity; and keeps blood clotting normally.

Iron is an abundant metal with many external uses and is a vital part of health of the human body. Iron is part of many enzymes and proteins as well as an essential component in transporting oxygen through the blood to all parts of the body. Heme iron and non-heme iron are the two dietary forms: heme iron is found in animal foods, and non-heme is found in plants and dairy products. Iron has a major role in producing energy as an essential element of several enzymes. The immune system is also dependent on sufficient levels of iron to function properly. Iron also aids in the production of carnitine, a substance that helps the body turn fat into energy. A healthy, balanced diet is imperative to keep iron levels normal.

Magnesium is a mineral that cannot be made by the body but is present in abundance in a variety of foods. Magnesium is found in the bones and teeth; because it aids in the absorption of calcium, it has a major role in their strength and formation. It also helps glands that regulate hormones important for bone health as well as a multitude of other functions. Magnesium helps turn our food into energy. The digestive system, cardiovascular system, nervous system, muscles, kidneys, liver, glands, and brain rely on its metabolic function. It helps stabilize the rhythm of the heart and blood pressure and aids in preventing blood clotting in the heart.

Manganese is a trace mineral that works with the enzyme systems and delivers alkaline buffers that neutralize acids in the body. The word *manganese* is derived from the Greek word for *magic*, which is very appropriate for this essential mineral. The healing process in the body is very complex, and manganese is required to start the process of healing. It helps maintain normal blood-sugar levels and strong bones, and it protects the cells and nerves from free-radical damage.

Potassium is the third most abundant mineral in the body and, along with sodium and chloride, belongs to the electrolyte family of minerals. These minerals conduct electricity when dissolved in water; thence, low electrolytes, lights out! Sorry, I couldn't help myself. Potassium's most important function is to take on a positive or negative charge to regulate blood pressure, which generally keeps our bodily functions working properly. Potassium is vital to maintain a good pH balance in the body and to protect against heart disease and stroke.

The message we may have missed in eighth grade science class is that the body can only utilize minerals if they come through the process of photosynthesis. The raw minerals must have been absorbed through a plant's growth process in order to be utilized and absorbed by the human body for nutrition. Raw minerals and metals are toxic and cause health deterioration.

Green vegetables, like broccoli, Brussels sprouts, spinach, kale, chard, asparagus, cucumber, and beans, are good sources of the primary alkaline minerals. These foods have a high alkalizing effect on the body and play a very important role in a balanced, healthy diet. There is really no perfect replacement for regularly eating the food sources that best support the primary minerals. However, some people dislike the foods that provide the essential minerals, and if this is the case, they can at least supplement with a good-quality, whole-food, multi-mineral supplement—along with healthy natural salts as these provide essential minerals as a replacement for table salt. The body needs minerals, including sodium, to break down and assimilate food.

Ordinary table salt, sodium chloride, is also a mineral. Salt is a necessary nutrient, but very little is needed, especially not ordinary table salt as it contains anticaking agents. More about healthy salts is covered in chapter 11, "Salts and Hydration."

Too much commercial sodium in the diet can contribute to harmful effects on health, like high blood pressure, heart failure, stroke, osteoporosis, stomach cancer, kidney malfunction, and disease. The problem is that the Western diet, or American diet, contains huge amounts of commercial sodium.

The average American should cut his or her sodium intake by more than half (to less than 1,500 milligrams a day). If Americans made this one change, the health-care system in the United States would save billions of dollars a year. That's why I strongly encourage you to eliminate processed and packaged foods; learn new ways to eat foods close to their natural state, using simple recipes and techniques; eat foods high in the primary minerals, especially potassium as it counters the effects of sodium; supplement with plant-based minerals; and use Himalayan sea salt, Celtic sea salt, Real Salt, or salt substitutes instead of ordinary table salt.

The good news is that it's easy to make the change. People worry that being healthy means sprouts and tofu. The idea of making drastic changes in the diet makes it seem impossible, but there are so many great foods that are alkaline or neutral that will support health and wellness. Included at the end of this chapter is an alkaline-acid food chart. It is a list of foods that are alkaline, neutral, or acidic. Dramatic, positive changes in health can be experienced by merely eating 75 percent alkaline and 25 percent acidic foods as the makeup of any meal or snack. Envision the dinner plate with three quarters of the plate filled with alkaline-forming food choices and one quarter of the same plate with acid-forming food choices. In addition, seasoning with herbs, spices, and healthy sea salt provides a huge health benefit for digestion and the absorption of vitamins and nutrients; plus, it gives a boost to the immune system.

Poor food choices are just one factor that causes our blood to lose an alkaline balance. Stress, anxiety, depression, sleep deprivation, and pollution can also contribute to a highly acidic pH level. A consistent alkaline-acid balanced diet will slowly correct these disturbances. I have seen many quickly improve their health situation with this awareness and a few simple changes. I follow this balance pretty closely because I believe it keeps me healthy and helps compensate for the stress in my life as well as the pollutants in my environment.

Just a little more science to provide a well-rounded view of the life-saving benefits of an alkaline diet: now that we have discussed the right minerals and how important they are to the overall operation of the body, where they come from, and how we improve and maintain our health with them, we also need to focus on how the minerals and nutrients are taken from our food by the body and absorbed for nutritional healing and overall health.

In the intestines, there are very small, slender, fingerlike projections along the lining that absorb nutrients from food as it goes by. These tiny projections are called villi (pronounced "vill-eye"). On the villi are smaller, hairlike villi called microvilli, which provide even more surface, or absorption area, for the nutrients to be received. Yes, that's right; we all have villi on our villi. The villi provide the avenue for the nutrients, vitamins, and minerals to be collected and absorbed from the food. When the body has been exposed to an unhealthy, acid-forming diet and other negative factors for health, the villi can become damaged. This doesn't allow the absorption of the products of food. Deficiency of vitamins, minerals, and nutrients in the diet and from malabsorption by the villi leads to a variety of illnesses and weakens our organs and the body's ability to make enzymes and hormones.

This is really where it all begins. I have witnessed the most gravely ill individuals turn their health around and move toward wellness by this simple, necessary change in their eating habits. It's the basic premise in nutrition that will slow aging, increase energy and vitality, and support weight loss and weight maintenance. It will also support healing and repairing the body back to wellness from cancer and cancer treatments, diabetes, and other illnesses, including inflammatory diseases.

Red and Steve lived a few miles from my home and were referred to me. While visiting with them the first day, Steve shared with me some of his medical problems. At the time, a friend of mine, a nutritional healing advisor who works with live-blood analysis, and I were about to give a series of nutritional healing classes in the next town, so I invited Steve and Red to sign up. They were a joy to share information with because they were like sponges, soaking up the information presented with enthusiasm. They set out to implement the basics for nutritional healing in their own lives. Since then, they have enjoyed much improvement in their health. Recently, with the sale of their home behind them, they moved across the country, and Steve sent this short story about his healing for me to share:

> *I met Donna through her work and found her passion was making people feel better by eliminating what they do not need in their body and increasing what they do need to live a healthy life. Once we started to eat foods that were less acidic and were more alkaline based, our outlook and health improved. If I slipped on our new diet and ate out of the alkaline group of foods, I would feel so sluggish as though I was not burning on all cylinders.*

There are many ways to support healing in the body. Understanding alkalinity and applying this knowledge is vital, and the result is tremendous and quick. The gift of natural enzymes in this process is vital as well, and the next chapter clears up the mystery behind living foods, healing energy, and vitality.

	HIGHLY	MODERATELY	MILDLY
ALKALINE	Baking Soda Broccoli Cucumber Grasses Green drinks Herbs (green) Himalayan Sea Salt Kale Kelp Lemons Limes Millet Mineral Water Nectarine Onion Parsley Pumpkin Seed Raspberries Sea Vegetables (Kelp) Spinach Spirulina Sprouted Beans/Sprouts Sprouts (soy, alfalfa etc.) Sweet Potato Tangerine Watermelon	Almonds Apples Avocado Beetroot Blackberry Blueberry Butter Beans Cabbage Capsicum/Pepper Celery Chia/Salba Collard/Spring Greens Endive Garlic Ginger Green Beans Lettuce Millet Mustard Greens Okra Pineapple Radish Red Onion Rocket/Arugula Spices Tomato	Apple Cider Vinegar Artichokes Asparagus Avocado Oil Brussels Sprouts Buckwheat Carrot Cauliflower Chives Coconut Coconut Oil Courgette/Zucchini Flax Oil Goat & Almond Milk Grapefruit Leeks Lentils New Baby Potatoes Other Beans & Legumes Peas Quinoa Rhubarb Spelt Strawberry Tofu Watercress

	MILDLY	MODERATELY	HIGHLY
ACIDIC	Amaranth Black Beans Brazil Nuts Cantaloupe Chicken Chickpeas/Garbanzos Currants Eggs Figs Fresh Dates Freshwater Wild Fish Gelatin Grapeseed Oil Hazel Nuts Honey Kidney Beans Maple Syrup Oats/Oatmeal Pecan Nuts Pine Nuts Plum Rice & Soy Milk Rice/Soy/Hemp Protein Seitan Spelt Soybeans Sunflower Oil Sweet Cherry	Apricot Banana Brown Rice Butter Cottage Cheese Cranberry Fresh, Natural Juice Grapes Ketchup Lard Mango Mangosteen Mayonnaise Ocean Fish Orange Papaya Pasta Peach Rye Bread Safflower Oil Tapioca Turkey Wheat Wholemeal Bread Wild Rice Yogurt (plain)	Alcohol Artificial Sweeteners Beef Brown Sugar Cheese Cocoa Coffee & Black Tea Dairy Dried Fruit Farmed Fish Fruit Juice (sweetened) Jam Jelly Miso Mushroom Mustard Pork Rice Syrup Shellfish Soy Sauce Soft Drinks Syrup Table Salt White Bread Wine Yeast Yogurt (sweetened)

Chapter 5
THE GIFT OF ENZYMES

Today you can change your health in a positive direction by simply eating something live every time you have a meal or snack. Enzymes are the most essential component of our bodies. Enzymes help us breathe, drink, eat, and digest.

Enzymes are present in uncooked food. Once food has been cooked, the high temperature destroys the enzymes. Raw foods (foods that are alive or the "live" component of your meal) contain enough natural food enzymes to digest food. When cooked, the enzymes in food are inactivated and can no longer assist the body in digestion. Eating raw food is easiest with vegetables and fruit. Nuts, dairy, sushi, and some meats are served raw or rare, which is also helpful.

There are three main categories of enzymes: (1) digestive enzymes, (2) food enzymes, and (3) metabolic enzymes. We are going to concentrate on the first two. There are three main types of digestive enzymes: (1) protease, (2) amylase, and (3) lipase. Each one has a different food component that it breaks down. Protease breaks down proteins, amylase breaks down carbohydrates, and lipase breaks down fats (also called lipids).

The body does produce the enzymes we just covered, but here's the problem: the body doesn't create an infinite amount of enzymes. We lose digestive enzymes through body waste, sweating, and other functions of the body that naturally work to stabilize, detoxify, and repair. So the strength and ability of the enzymes to do their work declines. In the processes of aging or with a lifestyle of poor eating habits, the body becomes less efficient in producing digestive enzymes. Processed food, microwave cooking, and environmental pollution can cause free radicals that lower the body's ability to produce enzymes as well.

Aging accelerates when the diet is short of, or missing, enzymes. The body cannot keep up with the demand, so acid reflux, indigestion, and bloating become prevalent issues. In order to support your body's natural process of ingesting, digesting, and repairing and regenerating healthy cells, two easy changes can be made to your diet.

First, eat a "live" food as part of every meal. Ultimately, minimize cooked food or at least cut back on cooked food portions and increase your raw components. Give the body a break and a much-needed boost to support the natural healing process and slow aging. Second, faithfully take a good digestive enzyme supplement to aid in the digestion of all foods. Make sure the digestive enzyme supplement has the three main digestive enzymes we reviewed (protease, amylase, and lipase). If you are treating an autoimmune or inflammatory disease, protease, which enables protein digestion, is imperative. Protease is often used as a separate therapy as it alleviates autoimmune and inflammatory conditions as well as pain.

Many believe they eat fairly well yet still have digestive problems. If digestion isn't happening properly, undigested food can seep into the bloodstream, which causes the immune system to react. There are many symptoms that provide evidence that a simple digestive enzyme is needed. For starters, discomfort and lack of energy may be present, but there are others to consider: arthritis, bloating, constipation, cravings, diarrhea, dull or thinning hair, depression, headaches, heartburn, hives, gas, rashes, and weak and cracked nails.

If the body is not functioning properly for any reason, taking digestive enzymes is easy and makes good sense. It will take a huge burden off the body and allow more nutrients to be broken down from food to promote healing and produce more energy. Once the body is digesting properly, the body needs less food because nutrients are readily absorbed; therefore, less food needs to be consumed.

Plant-based digestive enzymes are safe for adults and children. Adults should take digestive enzymes immediately before each meal. For children, taking a digestive-enzyme formula twice a day with a meal is good. Simply adding enzymes to a health regimen can dramatically change life for the better. It's so exciting, isn't it?

Digestive enzymes are found in humans, animals, and carnivorous plants as well as inside every cell. In the cell, the function of enzymes is to maintain the survival of the cell. Salivary glands secrete digestive enzymes, which is why it's so important to slow down and chew, chew, chew our food. The cells in the lining of the stomach, pancreas, and glands in the small intestine also secrete digestive enzymes.

Some examples of other digestive enzymes are galactosidase, which digests the starches that are hard to digest; cellulose, which aids in digestion of the cellulose fiber in fruits, grains, seeds, and vegetables; glucoamylase, which helps digest maltose, the sugar in grains; invertase, which aids in the digestion of sucrose (sugar); lactase, which digests lactose, or milk sugar; and peptidase, which helps digest casein in milk, gluten in grains, and pectin in fruits. Believe it or not, there are more, but the point is that enzymes cover a lot of bases in assisting the body in digesting and utilizing fats, proteins, sugars, and starches from food.

So, down to the facts: If we don't get enough raw foods and we don't eat slowly and chew food well, the body can't make enough enzymes to make up the difference. It's important to do these things, and if you have any symptoms or are experiencing illness or disease, you should also take digestive enzymes for the optimum digestion of food.

Some foods aggravate the body, cause inflammation, and are difficult to digest, and they cause disease. Incredibly, one of these is wheat. Many think patients suffering with celiac disease are the only ones affected by the ingestion of wheat. This could not be further from the truth. Wheat is a hot topic in the nutritional healing world and rightfully so. In the next chapter, I will shed some light on the subject to increase awareness of this genetically modified food and the mayhem it is causing.

Chapter 6
WHEAT AWARENESS

There is such a buzz about gluten right now, and most people say, "What the heck is gluten?" and "Why do we want to be free of it?" Yes, gluten is one of the culprits in the current health crisis. Gluten (from Latin meaning "glue") is a protein found in foods processed from wheat and related grains, including barley, rye, spelt, kamut, and some oats. Oats can be tricky because of processing; if you use oats, make sure they are specifically gluten-free or steel-cut oats. The stored proteins of corn and rice are sometimes called glutens, but their proteins differ and are not the health concern that is found in wheat.

Gluten is what gives elasticity to dough; it helps the dough to rise, helps keep its shape, and gives it a chewy texture. The more gluten is refined, the chewier the product, such as pizza and bagels; in contrast, less refining yields tender baked goods, such as pastry products. Generally, bread flours are high in gluten, while pastries are low in gluten.

Gluten is also used as a stabilizing agent in products like ice cream, ketchup, beer, and soy sauces. Foods made with wheat are staples in many diets; however, many people suffer the effects of wheat proteins that can cause chronic and acute illnesses. Upset stomach, bloating, eczema, allergic rhinitis, bronchospasm, and anaphylaxis are a few of the more common side effects of a gluten-heavy diet. Often, gluten in wheat is associated with celiac disease, so it is overlooked as a source of other illnesses. Conditions that make our lives a bit unpleasant, flare-ups followed by low-grade discomfort, leave many just accepting their body's state as a way of life—without hope of resolution. But these are all indications that something is not acceptable to the complex, intricate, biochemical operation of the body.

The truth is that gluten causes inflammation in 80 percent of the population. That is the big mayday sign. Things start going wrong, maybe a little sign here and there, then—*bang!*—some major medical condition presents itself. Gluten has been associated with cancer and other inflammatory and autoimmune diseases. *But*—and it's a big *but*—there is more to this story. Being gluten free is not the only reason for being wheat free. Some believe there is actually another protein that's a wicked villain in the story of wheat in addition to the gluten protein. It is the gliadin protein.

According to Dr. William Davis, a cardiologist who in 2011 published a book called *Wheat Belly* about the world's popular grains, "Modern wheat is a perfect chronic poison." If you love history too, this is an excellent book. The reason Dr. Davis and others make such extreme statements regarding wheat is because, like many good, old-fashioned ingredients, wheat has become commercially improved for the marketplace. I call it the "new and improved" syndrome. Wheat today is not the same wheat that our ancestors and grandparents enjoyed; it was genetically modified just a few decades ago. The new features that were added have major negative effects on everyone.

Gliadin protein is one of the worst offenders. It acts as an opiate in the brain. Opioid peptides found in wheat are known to cause addiction to wheat as well as withdrawal symptoms when wheat is removed from the diet. Gliadin binds in the opiate receptors in the brain and stimulates appetite. Hence, we want to eat more wheat.

Commercially, genetically modifying the wheat was smart and good business. It produced a much larger yield because gluten made the bud of the wheat fuller, and increased gliadin meant increased cravings. This created more demand. Statistics show the decline of health and increase of cancer, diabetes, and obesity in the past few decades—no coincidence here.

The findings are major. It's not just a handful of folks losing a few pounds. People who turn away from wheat are experiencing needed weight loss; however, they are also experiencing recovery from diabetes, acid reflux, irritable bowel syndrome, leaky gut syndrome, depression, and dramatic relief from arthritis. Basically, any inflammatory condition will find relief with the elimination of wheat.

Some people find these discoveries infuriating, to think of how much suffering that gliadin modification has caused and to know it was done deliberately. Observing a continued decline in the health of our population, especially in our youth, and the skyrocketing cost of medical treatment, it has led me to believe and accept that our food sources have been altered purely for economic gain, with no consideration of nutritional value. Today there are standards for genetically modifying foods, and it's done for a multitude of reasons. When the wheat modifications were done in the 1960s and 1970s, there were no standards and, I'm sure, no way of guessing how it would affect future generations.

Personally, I have been gluten free and, therefore, gliadin free for a long time and feel so much better. I have no problem controlling my weight. I didn't have a disease, but I did have a chronically stuffy nose, postnasal drip, and a bloated stomach. When I decided to remove wheat from my diet, these issues simply went away. I had read so many things about gluten over the years that I decided, why chance it? It was an easy decision and transition.

There are so many wonderful, gluten-free products on the market now that are very tasty, so it's not the struggle that it used to be to make the change. Ordinary foods like corn and rice are gluten free as well and can be easily substituted. Negative things about gluten and gliadin are very eye-opening; it's worth eliminating them to have the best chance possible to turn illness around and enjoy better health overall.

Making simple dietary changes, removing inflammatory foods like wheat, and adding anti-inflammatory foods like coconut, can cause dramatic, remarkable improvements to health. In the next chapter, I will look at some incredible findings about coconut.

Chapter 7
FINDING CURES
WITH COCONUTS

L ike a lot of things in the past, coconut oil got a bad rap for being a saturated fat. This was back when scientists thought that there was only one kind of cholesterol. There is good cholesterol (HDL) and bad cholesterol (LDL), and coconut oil actually aids in bringing cholesterol to healthy levels. Back then, the population scurried to get coconut oil out of the diet, just when the market was unwittingly introducing more destructive, inflammatory foods. Now as more studies have been completed, coconut has been found to have huge importance in our diet as a nutritional healing and antiaging aid. The body produces cholesterol naturally to protect our arteries from damage caused by free radicals and inflammation. The body produces more cholesterol when stressed, and because of this, cholesterol levels typically rise with age.

In the tropics where coconuts grow naturally as well as commercially, they have always been used as food and medicine. Recently, they have been rediscovered by the masses, and the healing qualities of coconut are a topic in every current natural-health information source.

The truth is that coconuts taste good and have a multitude of healing, antifungal, antibacterial, and anti-inflammatory properties. For those who don't like the taste of coconut, the more refined forms mean less coconut taste, but nutritional value is still present. Coconut oil can be used internally and externally. The popularity of treating everything from Alzheimer's to acne has created a worldwide buzz. There are testimonials around the globe of the quick, positive effect on overall health and illnesses when coconut oil, a medium-chain triglyceride, is applied or consumed for improved well-being.

Medium-chain triglycerides (MCTs) absorb into the digestive system and do not need bile salts for digestion; therefore, no modification is required. This is particularly important in ill patients with malnutrition or malabsorption as MCTs don't require energy for absorption or utilization. The three fatty acids that make up this triglyceride are capric acid, caprylic acid, and lauric acid.

Capric acid is a medium-chain fatty acid found in saturated fats. Found in coconut oil and a small amount in goat's milk and cow's milk, capric acid has antiviral and antimicrobial properties. It works with caprylic acid and lauric acid to raise good cholesterol (HDL) and lower bad cholesterol (LDL). HDL protects children from infections. It has been discovered that children with infections have high LDL.

Caprylic acid is an antifungal, short-chain fatty acid naturally derived from coconut and palm oil and is used to treat fungus and yeast infections caused by *Candida albicans*. Caprylic acid is quickly absorbed by the body, so if supplemented in the diet for the purpose of treating fungus, it should be taken with meals and essential oils, such as flaxseed oil or fish oil, and as a time-released formula to distribute it throughout the intestinal tract.

Lauric acid is a medium-chain fatty acid found in coconut oil. When lauric acid is in the body, it acts as an antiviral, antimicrobial, antifungal, and antiprotozoan agent. Lauric acid accomplishes this by disrupting the membrane in organisms like fungi, viruses, and bacteria, which destroys them. Since pure coconut oil contains about 50 percent lauric acid, it makes sense that using coconut oil would reduce the risk of illness and provide protection to the body while trying to recover from a disease.

Another source of MCTs is palm-kernel oil. Palm-kernel oil and palm oil both come from palm trees but differ in that the palm kernel is extracted from the seed and palm oil comes from the fruit. Palm-kernel oil is a healthy saturated fat as it also helps with total-cholesterol-to-HDL ratio.

Many illnesses are tied to inflammation, so it's important to offer the body a nutritional aid to keep the ratio of good and bad cholesterol in check. Coconut oil tends to be more popular as coconut is a treat to most people, is easy to find in grocery stores, is great for cooking or frying, and is desirable as a replacement for skin lotions.

The body is made of fifty trillion to one hundred trillion cells that provide energy to the body. People who are weak from an illness and others who just want to lose weight can benefit from the ability of the ketones in coconut oil to enter the cells and provide energy. Coconut oil is not stored by the body but is metabolized directly through the liver.

When glucose levels are unstable or nutrition for energy is not getting to the cells, the cells starve and die prematurely. If the body is not working properly, supplementing the diet with coconut oil allows MCTs to enter the cells without any special receptors. This happens without the aid of insulin, so cells get nutrients, even in a diabetic. Significant improvement can be made to health once the cells receive an easily absorbed energy source, such as coconut oil.

In researching coconut oil, I found that there is a lot of information available showing significant improvement for some patients with Alzheimer's. Dr. Mary Newport's work with coconut oil for her husband, Steve, who had Alzheimer's disease, is very impressive. Dr. Newport's 2011 book, *Alzheimer's Disease, What If There Was a Cure? The Story of Ketones,* has opened my mind about the possibilities of reversing this disease and expanded my thinking about coconut oil as an effective nutritional tool for improving memory as well as getting nutrition to cells when digestion is not functioning properly.

My goal is to provide some new insight into natural-food resources being used to support health recovery. Coconut oil definitely deserves its own space. I have read so much on the subject of coconut oil and find much information on its use for improving acne; acid reflux; arthritis; bedsores, burns, cold sores, dry skin, and other skin-related problems; thyroid conditions; fibromyalgia; yeast infections; cholesterol ratios; blood pressure; weight loss; dementia; multiple sclerosis; and the list goes on. It's a food, not a drug, so it's safe. The take-home message is, it's certainly worth the effort to learn as much as possible about this natural healing source and to incorporate it into the diet.

Chapter 8
GETTING BETTER WITH SLEEP

And now the tough principle for many people: we must sleep. Yes, we all need good old-fashioned rest. They say six to eight hours of sleep is good. You need a deep sleep to heal, detoxify the body, regenerate cells, slow down aging, and think clearly.

There is so much information out there today on sleeping because of its importance to our health and well-being. Sleep clinics have cropped up all over in the last decade to study our sleep habits and find solutions for this problem that makes all aspects of life difficult.

When I was young, I loved to stay at my grandmother's house. Everything was so fun and magical. Even when it was time for bed, we wouldn't just go to bed; we would sit and enjoy our sleeping potion that Grandma made in her lovely teacups. It was part milk and water warmed with a hint of nutmeg and a pinch of sugar. She would turn the small lamp on by the bed, then start to read a storybook. I always thought the potion worked great because just minutes after I lay down to hear the story, it was morning.

In that tale are some old remedies for sleep: a warm drink, a cozy setting, an easy book, and some loving care. This might truly be the best medicine, but in my research, I have found more possibilities to try.

Lifestyle and diet can cause the body's natural calming and excitement mechanism to be out of sync. The fight-or-flight response and the production of adrenaline and cortisol hormones in the body are normal for situations that require heightened awareness to respond immediately to danger. Unfortunately, this response and the resulting production of these hormones can become imbalanced and in some cases lead to adrenal failure when extreme stress continues for very long periods of time. Stress raises our blood pressure and body temperature and gets our muscles ready for action. Fortunately, we also produce chemicals that calm down our brain and nervous system which helps us to relax. These are neurotransmitters like GABA and serotonin. If there is an imbalance, chances are that you will not be able to calm down enough to go to sleep or stay asleep through the night.

In studies, people with sleep problems had the highest levels of cortisol in their bloodstream, especially in the evening. So if you need to improve your sleep, you must decrease your cortisol. Exercise helps and so does yoga or meditation, warm baths in some Epsom salts, soft music, or a quiet, dark bedroom with no electronics.

There are many supplements that can help. I will describe several natural sleep aids. All have been shown to help individuals relax, ease stress, and sleep better. You can experiment and see which ones might work best for you.

Serotonin is your body's "feel good" neurotransmitter. It helps to regulate your appetite and mood as well as your sleep. If you crave sweets and high-glycemic carbohydrates like cookies, crackers, and potato chips, then you might be deficient in serotonin. During the day, your body slowly converts serotonin into melatonin. Your body stores this melatonin in your pineal gland. At night, it signals your pineal gland to release the melatonin. The melatonin helps you fall asleep. If your serotonin levels are too low during the daytime, your melatonin levels will be too low at night.

Melatonin is a hormone secreted by the pineal gland in the brain that helps regulate sleep and wake cycles. Synthetic melatonin has been especially helpful to shift workers, sleeping in the daytime and working at night. It can be taken as a supplement, and you can purchase it without a prescription at health food stores, drugstores, and online. Side effects of melatonin include sleepiness, morning grogginess, vivid dreams, lower body temperature, and small changes in blood pressure. In adults, melatonin is taken in doses from 0.2 to 20.0 milligrams, based on the reason for its use. The right dose varies widely from one person to another. Talking to a doctor will help you find the right dosage.

Green tea has also been used as a bedtime tea because it contains L-theanine, an amino acid that stops the stimulating effects of caffeine and has an overall calming effect. L-theanine is like getting a short meditation session for calming your mind and promoting a deep and restful sleep.

Calcium is a very important mineral that works as a sleep aid, and you should make sure you have it in abundance, either in your diet or as a supplement every day. Calcium strengthens your teeth and bones, supports normal blood clotting and healthy heart function, is necessary for the contraction and relaxation of your muscles and blood vessels, and regulates body fluids (hormones and enzymes). Calcium can be found in milk, yogurt, cheese, tofu, refried beans, white/navy beans, agar, almonds, sesame, sardines, salmon, oats, turnip greens, broccoli, bok choy, spinach, oranges, and spices, such as dried and fresh basil, savory, marjoram, dill weed and seed (fresh or dried), thyme, parsley, sage, spearmint, and oregano.

Magnesium is needed for calcium to be absorbed. It's a delicate balance, and you surely must make sure you are getting both. Magnesium is a good choice for people who experience muscle aching and leg cramps as a disturbance to their rest. It's also a natural muscle relaxant and sedative. Symptoms of magnesium deficiency may include agitation and anxiety, restless leg syndrome (RLS), sleep disorders, irritability, abnormal heart rhythms, and low blood pressure. Rich sources of magnesium include legumes, green leafy vegetables, Brazil nuts, almonds, cashews, blackstrap molasses, pumpkin and squash seeds, pine nuts, and black walnuts. Other good dietary sources of this mineral include peanuts, beet greens, spinach, pistachio nuts, bananas, baked potatoes (with skin), chocolate, and cocoa powder. Many herbs, spices, and seaweeds supply magnesium, such as agar seaweed, coriander, dill weed, celery seed, sage, dried mustard, basil, cocoa powder, fennel seed, savory, cumin seed, tarragon, marjoram, and poppy seeds.

My coworker's wife had finished treatment for breast cancer and found that she was having a very difficult time getting to sleep. When she did finally fall asleep, it would be for a short time. I gave her some information from two different journals on melatonin, and she decided to try it. She was finally able to get some rest. It was like a miracle for her, but it is a very individual thing. I have had other people tell me that they tried melatonin and it didn't work for them. Others have said they had wild dreams but increased the dose a small amount and then it worked fine. Others have found relief by supplementing with a quality magnesium or taking magnesium and melatonin before bed. Keep searching until you find the right solution. Not sleeping properly is not an option. Sleeping is as important as any other part of the natural healing process.

A good way to reverse a serotonin deficiency is to take a natural amino acid called 5-HTP (5-hydroxytryptophan). Supplementing this amino acid increases your serotonin quickly because it is a precursor to the neurotransmitter, the final step in your body's process for the production of serotonin. Many studies have shown that 5-HTP decreases the time needed to fall asleep and reduces the number of nighttime awakenings. It also increases your REM sleep and boosts your deep, restorative sleep.

Supplementing with vitamin B will boost serotonin, too. Vitamin B-3 (niacinamide) is a potent sleep aid and helps the body make neurotransmitters like serotonin; also, vitamin B-6 (pyridoxine) helps the body minimize the effects of stress and is also essential in creating serotonin. Personally, I have always been a good sleeper, but I have supplemented with B vitamins for many decades. I take B-100, a complex of the Bs, and earlier in my life, I used a vitamin called Stress Life that was a vitamin B complex, with a little different structure and potency. Both worked well for me. I will add that B vitamins are better to take during the day with food. They help you sleep better at night because they give you more energy, so you do more and have a better chance of getting sleep.

Last but not least is exercise. A walk is a wonderful thing. It helps create more energy and the ability to sleep better. Go first thing in the morning, on your lunch break, or after dinner. Breathe, clear your mind, enjoy the view, and get your blood moving.

Chapter 9
RELEASING THOSE STRESSFUL THOUGHTS AND FEELINGS

When I meet with someone who is ill, he is generally filled with stressful thoughts because a doctor has told him that he has precancerous cells, cancer, or some other debilitating illness or disease. I believe that the hormones created by stress actually create a better environment for illness or disease to spread and flourish. The production of cortisol and adrenaline, your fight-or-flight response when you are stressed, creates a huge amount of havoc in your body. A chronically high cortisol level interferes with digestion, immune function, sleep, and the body's ability to produce other essential hormones, such as DHEA, testosterone, estrogen, progesterone, and thyroid hormone. Over time, unrelenting cortisol production can contribute to excess abdominal fat, high blood pressure, high blood sugar, and aches and pains from too much inflammation. It demands too much from the adrenal glands and affects DHEA production, which, in turn, compromises bone health, immunity, mood, and sex drive.

When the adrenal glands become compromised, it's harder for them to make cortisol. Instead, extra adrenaline is produced to compensate, which can make you irritable, shaky, and downright mean. Adrenal fatigue can cause low blood sugar, anxiety, inability to concentrate, light-headedness on standing, allergies, and low blood pressure. This contributes to those bouts of total exhaustion that eventually become a way of life for some.

The good news is that this pattern can be reversed, and yes, it is a pattern of thinking. Through better diet, the reduction of stress-related areas of your life, and becoming more familiar with your emotional guidance system, you can change this pattern of destruction in your body.

Getting someone to visualize something bad happening in his body every time he dwells on fruitless thoughts and worry has been the easiest way for me to get him to stop in his tracks and change his thoughts. Since I have taught that an alkaline diet retards the growth of cancer cells and inflammation and that an acid environment is a perfect host for cancer cells and increases inflammation, I ask the individual to visualize a hose squirting acid into the body whenever he is stressing about something. This makes him keenly aware of the damage he is creating, and he immediately tries to change his state of thinking.

Using any technique you can find to get relaxed and to free yourself of bad thoughts is just as important as all the other things you might do for naturally getting yourself back to good health. Yes, I know you have received really bad news and your life is turned upside down. I have had it happen to me and my family and was forced to find healthy ways for us to cope.

When my daughter was going through her chemotherapy, it was mostly in-hospital, and she had to endure such difficult things that kids shouldn't have to know about. When she was going through a rough time, I would have her close her eyes, and I would guide her through a visualization that she loved. At the time, she loved horses and had taken riding lessons at a small farm that taught the young rider all aspects of horse care. When she arrived, she would walk up to the paddock and get her horse or try to catch one, depending on their mood, and bring it down to the barn and prepare it for riding. She would then tack up and head to the ring. After her lesson, she removed the tack and put it away, cleaned her horse, and took him back to the field; then she mucked out a few stalls before I arrived to pick her up.

I would create this scene for her in her mind; every detail that I could think of, I would describe to her so she could put herself there and change her thoughts about what was happening around her. She loved this, and it soothed her and calmed her down when nothing else helped. When I learned about this approach, I was mentally stuck and sad, and I was open to any suggestions to move me forward toward peace and to reunite me with happiness again.

Another great stress reducer is to talk with someone close or someone who has been through what you are experiencing so that you can verbalize your greatest fears and begin to work through them. I learned that there are many support groups out there for the most difficult illnesses. If there isn't one, you should start one in your area because you are definitely not suffering alone. I'm sure there is someone going through a similarly tough situation who wishes there was a support group that would help him through it. Even if you have trouble socializing and feel that a therapy group is not your thing, sometimes just going once allows you to meet someone that you resonate with, and then you can get together with that person independently of the group.

This happened to Monica and me when we were in the medical center for her treatment. The social worker kept coming in the room every other day or so, suggesting that Monica meet with other kids in the cancer wing and that I go to a parents' support group that met on Wednesdays. Monica and I both felt like we had each other and our family and friends for support and didn't need all these extra people, who were probably sad and sick. We didn't understand how outsiders could help us heal.

There was a point several months into the illness that things were really bad, and I said to Monica one morning, "Today is parents' support group; maybe I should go and see if there is something else we should consider trying to help you." She thought it might be a good idea too, so I went.

There were about six other parents and the social worker at the meeting. Everyone went around and said his name and told the story of his child's illness that had eventually brought him there. Everyone had a different type of cancer challenge, but that was our common link: parents with a child receiving some kind of cutting-edge cancer treatment. I bonded with a father who was there who had a thirteen-year-old daughter with several brain tumors. He explained that a side effect of one of her treatments caused leukemia. I was astounded and moved. Here we were, just dealing with leukemia, and he was looking at that as a potential side effect for his poor daughter. I took this story back to Monica; she wanted to go immediately and meet this girl. I loaded Monica in a wheelchair, and we headed to the end of the hall. There she was, lying in bed with bandages all over her head and covering one eye that had been damaged by the tumors. She and Monica became fast friends as I did with this sweet girl's mom and dad.

Back at home, a lovely woman I had met through a real estate transaction, Joanna, was doing a casual women's healing support group she called "Circle" in her home. I'm sure she had no idea how many lives she helped by offering this, but it had a wonderful chain effect. There were usually twelve to fifteen women who would come to her home. She held Circle the first Monday of each month at seven in the evening. The women would sit in a circle, and Joanna would lead with some nice thoughts she had or things she knew about in our town, and then she would turn to the person to her right and offer up the "talking stick." When you held the talking stick in Circle, you had the floor, and everyone else had to hush and listen to your story.

Your story could be whatever you were going through in life at the time or maybe some good things that had turned around for you. Sometimes new people felt awkward, so Joanna had cards spread on the floor in the center, facedown, that had different one-word topics on them, like truth, confidence, health, finance, love, guidance, etc., and you could pick a card and just tell what that card topic meant in your life. Women would meet new friends this way who had similar stories and would create new friendships outside of Circle. This was so popular and always well attended by new faces. Joanna is a nondenominational minister now and offers her support and loving guidance in a broader scope, but she still occasionally makes time for a Circle gathering.

There are so many tools that helped to guide me away from worrying and stressing. When my husband passed away, my friend Sybilla, a talented financial advisor by profession and a wonderful feng shui master by passion, offered to come to my home and create a *bagua,* a pattern determining the significance of spatial relationships, and change the energy of my home to help my daughter and me adapt to the sudden change. I was very familiar with feng shui and thought it to be an interesting approach to enhancing space. I had learned about this Eastern way of looking at energy because of my real estate practice as it is used commonly in the purchase, building, and decorating of homes and facilities, but I had personally never tried it.

I had been married for thirty-four years. We had bought that home twenty-eight years earlier, and it was also the place of my husband's home business. With his passing, the house seemed so different. Sybilla's offer to come three months after his passing seemed like just the right medicine. I was emotionally stuck and sad, but I was open to any suggestions to move me forward toward peace and to reunite with happiness again. Sybilla has suggested that I share from Eastern philosophy some of the basic feng shui elements for positive change that she uses with her clients. Here are eight ways to enhance your environment:

Assess Your Space

Stand back and look at your environment with a discriminating eye. Notice everything in each room and how you feel about it. This is a wonderful exercise for you to establish a connection to the room and how you feel about it, which either enhances your chi (energy) or creates negative chi (energy).

Clear Your Space

The art of space clearing has been with us for centuries. It involves the use of sound or clearing techniques to change the energy of a space.

Practice Intention Power

Now decide what you want to energize, and focus on how wonderful it will feel to have that come true, such as increased abundance, more love, and better health.

Create Space

Once you have thoroughly cleared and cleaned the area and stored anything that is not presently needed or used from this area, allow the space to be empty for a while. Nature abhors a vacuum, and before you know it, you will attract something representative in your life that will be of the intentional aspiration you wish to increase.

Reposition Artwork

Examine your artwork in every room. Do you love where it currently is? Try moving it around to different areas in your home. Pick something that reminds you of love, abundance, family, etc.

Bring in Living Chi (energy)

Enhance your space with living positive energy, such as with lovely plants. Add freshly cut flowers to a room for an instant refresher and energizer for the room.

Enhance Your Entrance

Notice the pathway to the front door. If it has any clutter or debris, clear it away. Add a fresh container of flowers at the door or a lovely wreath for the door with brightly colored silk flowers. You will instantly attract positive energy to your door and enjoy it in your home.

Sense for Scents

Notice the smells in your home or in the rooms. Is there anything unpleasant or stale? Scents have a powerful effect on us and can be uplifting to our emotions or help create negative emotions. Consider natural essential oils, such as citrus or lavender scents, for an overall clean and positive feeling. Aromatherapy is known to be a refreshing and stimulating healing aid to use in our homes and business. Have fun with it, and blend a scent that makes you feel alive and energized. (http://www.positivelivingfengshui. com/, accessed April 25, 2016)

My life has dramatically changed in so many ways since that first feng shui session six years ago. Recently I bought a new home that I could never have dared to dream of owning in the past, and Sybilla came through and applied her words of wisdom for having good energy and positive possibilities throughout my living space. I also have a new love in my life who has made all the difference in helping me get this work of healing out to the world. There is definitely something to this; you should try it!

There are many other healing approaches for stress, like massage, Reiki, pressure-point therapy, yoga, meditation, acupuncture, music therapy, deep-breathing routines, and exercise. Basically, anything that makes you feel the least bit better is worth trying. The bottom line is that the distraction of a different thought or activity is helpful to reduce worry and relieve stress, which are positive steps in the direction of healing.

Chapter 10
PROPER ELIMINATION

When I speak with someone about what to do to achieve an important edge while fighting an illness or disease, the topic of elimination is always discussed. Proper elimination is as important as a proper diet. I can't go on about what needs to go into the body without addressing how digested food needs to exit the body. Discreet parenting has led us to commonly call our toilet visits "number one" or "number two" to explain this personal task. So we will work on number two first then visit and gain knowledge of the importance of a good number one as well! We will then explore other means of elimination unique to the human body.

Many people have adjusted to constipation as a way of life, which is why so many people keep magazines and books in bathrooms. Your body is definitely sending you a very loud and specific message if you are constipated. Our bodies need fiber and a certain amount of fluid to operate properly. If we are not taking in enough fluid, our clever bodies will take fluid from our stool to circulate through our blood and organs in an effort to keep the heart beating. That's just bad news.

And then there are those of us who have never had constipation, but who also have never had a formed stool. That is just as bad. When eating and experiencing constant diarrhea, the body is not absorbing the necessary vitamins and nutrients from the food. What I have seen most often with patients taking a lot of medications for an illness is constipation lapsing into periodic diarrhea because of overcompensation of natural and medicinal laxatives. I worry that people are too private about this topic and let a potentially serious symptom, such as constipation or diarrhea, continue without taking any action.

There are two types of constipation: obstructed defecation and colonic slow transit. Causes of constipation include diet, hormones, side effects of medications, and heavy metal toxicity. Treatment includes changes in dietary habits, laxatives, enemas, biofeedback, and sometimes surgery. I believe that you should approach your illness proactively, especially when it comes to your daily elimination. The body has its own wonderful system of healing naturally if we give it the right things to work with. We eliminate toxins in more ways than toilet elimination. The body eliminates toxins through the kidneys, intestines, lungs, lymph nodes, and skin. When our system is compromised and impurities aren't properly filtered and eliminated, there is a negative effect on every cell. It may help if you fast for a day or two, juicing or just drinking healthy liquids or using your blender to add raw fruits (lemon, apple, berries, kiwi, etc.) and raw vegetables (parsley, cabbage, kale, cucumber, etc.) with water and some greens, hydrating yourself and providing nutrition at the same time. I personally like to add supplements to the drink, such as a scoop of powdered greens and probiotics, to help keep my intestinal tract healthy and absorbing nutrients properly. I also recommend drinking herbal teas throughout the day.

As you reintroduce solid foods, you may want to keep this daily practice going as a good and easy way to get some good nutrition in you first thing in the morning. You can add Greek yogurt to the drink to bring in your probiotics and protein for a better balance. Most people don't like the taste of greens or yogurt, but in this drink, they go unnoticed.

Be sure to clean your fruits and vegetables and to buy organic if at all possible, though I do realize that getting organic products is not easy or affordable for everyone. You can also use a nontoxic natural veggie wash (available in your grocery store, generally in the produce section) or white vinegar with plenty of rinsing before making your juice drink.

So let's get back to number two and what it should look like! Yes, there is a scale to measure this performance.

The Bristol stool scale is a medical aid designed to classify the form of human feces into seven categories. It was developed by Dr. Ken Heaton at the University of Bristol and was first published in 1997. It was his paper that concluded that the form of the stool is a useful surrogate measure of colonic transit time. It is still used as a research tool and clinical communication aid.

One and two indicate constipation, with three and four being the ideal stools (especially the latter) as they are easy to defecate while not containing any excess liquid. Five, six, and seven tend toward diarrhea. How often should you have a bowel movement? The answer may vary from person to person, but usually it depends on the number of meals you eat during the day. It's considered normal to have three bowel movements in a day if you eat two to three meals a day. At the very minimum, you should have one a day. In addition to your eating and drinking a good, healthy alkaline diet to improve elimination through bowel movements, it is also important to have good sleep and reduce stress.

Now let's consider number one in the toilet. Taking a look at urination with some basic knowledge helps one decide if the body function is normal or if there is need for diet or hydration change or a trip to the doctor. Urine appearance is a good natural diagnostic tool that is as old as time! It can reveal that you are dehydrated, have an infection, have taken a vitamin or medication, or have consumed a food tinted with color, naturally or dyed.

Normal can vary from individual to individual. No color can indicate too much drinking of water or maybe caffeinated beverages.

Bristol Stool Chart

Type 1	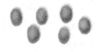	Separate hard lumps, like nuts (hard to pass) **Very Constipated**
Type 2		Sausage-shaped but lumpy **Slightly Constipated**
Type 3		Like a sausage with cracks on the surface **Normal**
Type 4		Like a sausage, smooth and soft **Normal**
Type 5		Soft blobs, clear cut edges (passes easily) **Lacking Fiber**
Type 6		Fluffy pieces, ragged edges, mushy stool **Inflammation**
Type 7		Watery, no solid pieces. Entirely liquid **Inflammation**

Deep shades of yellow can indicate dehydration. Cloudy urine can indicate phosphates, which could be an indication of kidney stones or an infection. If one experiences pain, urgency, or a burning sensation while urinating, this may require a trip to the doctor.

It's not uncommon for urine to pass in other shades of color. Blue to greenish urine may be a result of vitamins, laxatives, chemo drugs, or other medications. Orange urine can be an indication of vitamin B or vitamin C from supplements or food sources like carrots, beets, or citrus, although it can also occur from medications. Dark orange to brown urine can indicate that there is a problem with the liver or bile in the urine; both are cause for concern, requiring further testing by a doctor. Pink to red urine can simply indicate the consumption of red dye in foods or foods extremely red, like beets. It can also be a sign of blood in urine, which could occur from infections or a multitude of other medical conditions, requiring a visit with the doctor.

Urine can also smell sweet (not joking), foul, or musty. Sweet-smelling urine could be an indication of diabetes. Foul-smelling urine could be a sign of an infection or a particular food consumption, such as asparagus, and musty-smelling urine can be an indication of metabolic disorder or liver disease.

It's good to know the tendency toward normal for proper elimination of number one and two, but there are more ways the body eliminates in order to detoxify. Another source of natural elimination is breathing. For thousands of years, cultures have used breathing as a powerful tool to detoxify the body and overcome blues, stress, and depression. Proper breathing techniques are taught by instructors of every fitness and relaxation class. It is so important to overall health and clarity that no instructor will miss the opportunity to remind you to breathe. I think it's especially important to get you to incorporate a habit of being mindful about your breath a few times a day, especially whenever you need to calm yourself down.

There are so many great techniques out there. One I like is mind-detox breathing. It is very simple. You sit in a comfortable position with your spine erect. You can sit cross-legged or in any position that you feel comfortable. Breathe normally for about a minute. Then once you are composed, begin to exhale suddenly and quickly through both nostrils, producing a puffing sound, not focusing on inhalation. Inhalation will be automatic and passive. As the air is quickly exhaled completely with the sudden, vigorous puffs through the nose, your abdominal muscles will simultaneously draw inward and tighten. Once the breath is fully expelled, inhaling is automatic, and the abdominal muscles will automatically relax. Do the exercise in rounds of three, building up as you feel stronger and have more endurance.

This simple mind-detox breathing exercise has tremendous physical benefits to the digestive organs and circulatory system. It also helps you to feel totally de-stressed and calm with mental clarity. This technique tremendously increases the exchange of gases in the lungs. There is large-scale elimination of carbon dioxide and a huge absorption of oxygen, thus giving your body the precious gift of oxygen in your blood. Oxygen will rejuvenate energy and detoxify every cell, another amazing tool to healing naturally. This technique can be done while waiting at a red light, taking a walk, or before taking a rest. Making it a new habit can increase the speed of healing and reverse aging.

The lymphatic system is another way the body heals itself. Made up of the lymph nodes, spleen, thymus, and vessels that carry fluids that protect the body from disease and clean the individual cells, the lymphatic system can become sluggish and dysfunctional when we eat the wrong types of foods, if we don't exercise, or if we suffer from a prolonged illness. You can start out immediately improving your health by eating a diet of 75 percent to 80 percent alkaline foods. When your system is alkaline, your cells will float around freely and will file through the lymph nodes for cleaning. When your body is acidic, your cells clump together, not allowing for the natural cleansing and elimination to occur. This keeps your body in a dysfunctional state, leading to compromised cells, inflammation, and disease.

Good hydration, vegetables, fruits, and other stable, alkaline food choices will aid your body to heal itself and give you a better opportunity to reverse your illness. You should also consider an appointment with a lymphatic massage therapist; it is so important to pull out all the stops when you are sick and to take advantage of all the avenues to getting better.

The skin is another incredible part of our natural elimination system that is so perfect to help us retain good health. Taking a warm bath in Epsom salts (magnesium sulfate) has long been a way to soothe aches, soften skin, and possibly reduce wrinkles. Magnesium is important because it helps keep enzyme activity regular in the body. More than half of all Americans are magnesium deficient, which leads to a variety of health problems. Sulfate is also important, and it has a role in the formation of brain tissue, flushing out toxins, helping form protein in joints, and strengthening the walls of the digestive tract. If you are not physically able to use Epsom salts in a bathtub, use them in a footbath. Some doctors say to use them three times a week for up to thirty minutes of soaking. I know people who use a cup or two every day in their tub to detoxify and relax.

Reduce and eliminate the use of products with perfumes and possible toxic ingredients on your skin. Consider switching to a deodorant stone instead of commercial deodorants; after a few days with one of these natural stones you will be odor free and no longer applying harmful chemicals to your skin daily. Stick to oils like coconut oil to smooth into your skin after a bath or shower to hold in the moisture, and give yourself a nice helping of good fats that your body eagerly receives and knows how to use to balance your health. Also, using a natural sponge or loofah gloves to exfoliate your skin also enhances surface circulation. Removing dead skin not only improves the look of your skin, but it also cleans places that bacteria and soil could collect.

Keeping your skin clean and free of debris is just another way of eliminating toxins from your body and aiding the healing process. Many use a dry technique called skin brushing (also called dry-body brushing), which is a simple technique that stimulates blood flow, exfoliates the skin, and encourages new cell growth. This all may sound bad, but it feels good, which is another reason to try it. Improving circulation is an important component to improving health when faced with various illnesses. Everyone can benefit by exfoliation and skin brushing. I believe it is an exceptional way for pre-diabetics and diabetics to improve circulation and blood flow. A later chapter focuses on topics to support and improve the health of a diabetic and also contains information on stabilizing blood sugar.

Chapter 11

SALTS AND HYDRATION

There are many kinds of salt and many sources of salt, and the right salt is a critical part of the body's chemistry. Some sources are great or good; others are unhealthy and damaging to the body. The source of salt in the average diet is a problem that has caused major health issues. The increased salt-related health issues have led the population to turn away from all salt, which, in turn, also has a negative effect on health. So let's take a look at salt and what is considered the right salts for normal body functions.

Ordinary table salt, sodium chloride, is a mineral that does not support the body's overall health. Public awareness information has been relentless on the topic of reducing or eliminating the use of ordinary table salt. The body does need a balance of minerals, such as salts, but not table salt, so only part of the message has been loud and clear. The planet's salt comes from the oceans, lakes, and salt mines. In its natural state, salt is a combination of sodium, chlorine, and trace minerals. In the production of ordinary table salt, trace minerals are either removed for their commercial value or depleted in processing the salt at extremely high temperatures, up to 1200 degrees Fahrenheit in some cases. The sodium and chlorine (when combined, they are called sodium chloride), combined with anticaking agents, is sold as table salt.

A side note on anticaking and bleaching agents: You will see them in food and other products under a multitude of names such as silicoaluminate, fluoride, tricalcium phosphate, and manufactured forms of sodium aluminate. They make the sodium chloride white after it has been heated at extremely high temperatures. This also keeps it from caking so that it can flow freely when poured. The whole process removes more than eighty naturally occurring minerals and elements. It also bleaches, flakes, dries, and then fortifies the salt with synthetic iodine, producing ordinary table salt. Some companies also add sugar and MSG (monosodium glutamate) to the ingredient list of salt and salt substitutes.

Looking for a deeper explanation of anticaking agents, I turned to Wikipedia, my personal favorite. I was raised in the pre-computer era with Webster's dictionary and *World Book Encyclopedia* for the answers to most of the research in my youth. I found what Wikipedia had to say very interesting. Anticaking agents such as sodium aluminosilicate are manmade and are often used in nonfood items such as road salt, fertilizers, cosmetics, and detergents. Here's what Wikipedia said:

> An anti-caking agent is an additive placed in powdered or granulated materials, such as table salt, to prevent the formation of lumps and for easing packaging, transport, and consumption. An anti-caking agent in salt is denoted in the ingredients, for example, as "anti-caking agent labeled as (554)," which is sodium aluminosilicate, a man-made product. This product is present in many commercial table salts as well as dried milks, egg mixes, sugar products, and flours. In Europe, sodium ferrocyanide (535) and potassium ferrocyanide (536) are more common anti-caking agents in table salt. Natural anti-

caking agents used in more expensive table salt include calcium carbonate and magnesium carbonate.

Some anti-caking agents are soluble in water; others are soluble in alcohols or other organic solvents. They function either by absorbing excess moisture or by coating particles and making them water repellent. Calcium silicate (CaSiO3) is a commonly used anti-caking agent added to table salt; it absorbs both water and oil. (https://en.wikipedia.org/wiki/Anticaking_agent, accessed February 18, 2016)

Here are information and considerations of the side effects of anticaking agents from a popular health blog: "The most commonly used anti-caking agent is actually E554 sodium aluminosilicate. You guessed it! There can be side effects such as constipation along with many precautions if you have liver or kidney disease. E554 sodium aluminosilicate has many uses besides table salt. Did you know it is also added to road salt? Interesting!" (http://www.onlineholistichealth.com/truth-sea-salt/, accessed February 18, 2016)

Table salt contains processed sodium chloride fortified with synthetic iodine and anticaking food additives. Sea salt, on the other hand, comes from the ocean (as the name obviously implies) and naturally contains over fifty trace minerals, including natural iodine. The key here is the trace minerals that are found not only in our oceans but also in our soil. In fact, trace minerals are found in small amounts in our bodies. They are important for metabolic functions in the body. For example, if trace minerals are deficient in the body, then other substances and enzymes will not work properly. This could then impede major systems, such as the nervous system and musculoskeletal system. (Of course, these two systems are very important in chiropractic care.) Did you know that deficiencies in trace minerals, such as chromium and vanadium, may also play a major role in the development of diabetes? Other roles that trace minerals play in health care are as follows:

- Iodine, needed for thyroid function
- Iron, needed for blood-cell hemoglobin production
- Zinc, needed for normal immune function
- Chromium, needed for blood glucose and cholesterol metabolism
- Manganese and enzyme activation, needed in cell metabolism
- Boron, needed to prevent osteoporosis

Sea salt itself can be used to improve adrenal function and fatigue. Look for the phrase "50+ trace minerals" or more on sea salt to avoid purchasing unhealthy salt. Unfortunately, there are sea salt brands on the market that are indeed no healthier for you than regular salt. So how do you know if you have the real deal, meaning that it hasn't gone through the same extensive processing as table salt? Check it out; look at the color. It should not be white. Instead, it should have more of a pinkish or gray shade.

The body needs salt in its natural form: sodium chloride and minerals. In natural healing, natural, raw-harvested sea salt containing sodium chloride with natural primary and trace minerals is best. Sodium, potassium, magnesium, and other minerals have a salty taste. Often explained as pH salts, salt with minerals (or sea salts) are needed for the balance of the body's fluids, blood pressure, and blood volume in the circulatory system. Natural salts also keep the acid balance in check and aid in digestion. These minerals have many functions in balancing hormones, producing enzymes, and aiding organ function; they also have an alkalizing effect on the body. Properly balanced, they work in harmony to keep the complex chemistry of the body working properly. Sodium and chloride are not made by the body and must be provided in food. Sodium is a mineral that has critical functions within the body beyond regulating blood pressure and balancing acid. Sodium is also important for nerve transmission and the passage of nutrients into cells. Most of the body's sodium is in the organs, cells, blood, and extracellular fluids; the remainder is found in bones.

Chloride is a little harder to explain. The basic definition sounds like a bad day in chemistry class. Basically, the importance of chloride is balancing blood volume, blood pressure, muscle activity, and the pH balance of the body's fluids. Chloride ions are secreted as gastric juices in the stomach, called hydrochloric acid, a naturally produced acid critical for digestion. Chloride, sodium, and potassium in the body function as electrolytes. Electrolytes are particles that carry an electrical charge. The electrical charge carries nerve impulses, contracts muscles, and helps regulate heartbeat. Potassium is found in high concentration in cells. In addition to its work with sodium chloride for nerve and muscle function, it is also necessary for enzyme activity involved in metabolizing carbohydrates, changing food into forms that can be used by the body, and extracting energy for cell use.

The importance of electrolytes was driven home quite a few years ago in our little hometown. A prominent attorney in his early fifties who was known for being active and health conscious came home from the gym one day and had a heart attack and died. The autopsy said it was from an electrolyte imbalance. Intense exercise without proper salt, minerals, and hydration led to a sad and premature death for this great fellow. His story is what inspired me to give so much information in this chapter.

Salt and hydration seem basic, yet they are paramount in every fundamental approach to healing the body. Trace minerals are just as their name suggests: a very small amount of minerals or minor minerals. The body can utilize only minerals from plants. The body cannot absorb or utilize metallic minerals from the ground; the minerals must go through photosynthesis to be available to the body. Types of trace minerals are iron, cobalt, copper, fluoride, zinc, molybdenum iodine, chromium, and selenium. Although just a minute amount of these minerals is needed, it is still essential that the body gets them.

In the past, the trace minerals and essential minerals were easily part of our harvest of fruits and vegetables. It takes a full spectrum, the rainbow of food choices, eaten consistently to provide a good balance of vitamins and minerals. The new era of packaged, processed fast foods is deficient in the recommended daily intake of trace and essential minerals. This is where the argument for supplementing with a quality multi-mineral makes good sense. Becoming aware and enjoying the astounding health benefits of a diet rich in fresh, whole foods that provide all the vitamins and minerals is a huge step in health recovery, antiaging, and longevity. Part of a healthy eating plan includes substitutes for ordinary table salt. Using Himalayan sea salt, Real Salt, or Celtic salt will provide natural salt with the accompanying necessary minerals.

There are even more ways to naturally incorporate quality minerals into the daily diet regimen. For more flavor and tremendous health benefits, add more herbs and spices to your meals. There are generous amounts of minerals and vitamins in the most common herbs and spices. Commercial salt substitutes, like Chef Paul Prudhomme's Magic Salt-Free Seasoning, Spike® Salt-Free Magic!, and Mrs. Dash, or a popular hybrid sea salt/herb product like Herbamare (a blend of sea salt and fourteen organic herbs) will enhance the flavor of food while delivering healthy minerals and pH balance. We must not forget iodine. Humans need iodine for the normal metabolism of cells, the process of converting food into energy, and also for the production of thyroid hormones and normal thyroid function. So if you are using a replacement for table salt, be mindful of a source with natural iodine.

Another important thing to consider is that fluoride leaches iodine from the body; although we need a trace amount of fluoride, too much can remove essential iodine. Consideration must be given to the many sources of fluoride, such as in toothpaste, mouthwash, and public drinking water sources as they are fortified with fluoride. It's worth it to protect the thyroid by getting iodine from natural sources.

Over the years, I have enjoyed the natural salt, Himalayan sea salt, with a full array of trace minerals and natural iodine. This salt is pink in color and has all the natural elements identical to the elements in the body. This salt is raw harvested and not heated, and it is used entirely in its raw state from the earth. The body easily utilizes this pH-balanced source of sodium; it also enhances and brings out the full flavor of herbs and spices, with the added bonus of a beautiful natural color.

Let's next consider proper hydration. Don't go crazy on the salts and then forget to drink water. For an easy plan to support good hydration, fill a pitcher and put it in your refrigerator and make sure it's gone before you go to bed at night. Better yet, make the water alkaline by adding some lemons, limes, or both. Cucumbers are also a good addition as they leave the water tasting very fresh and also alkaline. This will detoxify the body while supporting the blood and fluids.

It's also easy to get great alkaline water by adding a pinch of baking soda (a brand without man-made anticaking agents, of course) or a pinch of Himalayan sea salt to drinking water to replace the body's natural saline fluid. This will provide a gentle pH-balance enhancement to regular drinking water, plus essential trace minerals. Another healthy choice for the kidneys and pH balance is a cup of warm water with a squeeze from a lemon before going to sleep or first thing upon waking. It's cleansing, relaxing, and nourishing at the same time.

The most common measure of proper hydration is half of your body weight in ounces of water intake. So, for example, if an individual's weight is 150 pounds, that person should drink a minimum of 75 ounces of water a day, which is roughly nine cups of water a day. Again, it is easier and better for the body to get this hydration with a pinch of sea salt with trace minerals so that the fluid being replaced has electrolytes and trace minerals similar to the natural fluid of the body. There are a few ways of looking to the body for clues of hydration or dehydration. If the tips of the fingers are wrinkled on the pads instead of plump and smooth, it could be dehydration. Headaches, yawning, fatigue, sunken eyes, and no tears can also be signs of dehydration. Constipation, as I mentioned earlier, is also another miserable sign of dehydration.

An easy way to monitor the body for dehydration is in the morning with the first urine elimination of the day. If it is light yellow like lemonade, you are hydrated; if you have dark urine and/ or urinate frequently, you are dehydrated. Dehydration can cause high blood pressure and dangerous low blood pressure in some individuals. Optimum Health Natural Healthcare Center, via the *Optimum Health* blog, has this to offer about dehydration and blood pressure:

Can Dehydration Cause High Blood Pressure?

Absolutely. Think of cooking oatmeal with plenty of water in the pot. Once the oatmeal is cooked, you can turn the pot upside down and the oatmeal will run out of the pot. Why? Because gravity is strong enough to pull the oatmeal from the pot. If you put too little water in the pot when cooking the oatmeal, the oatmeal will not run out of the pot when you turn it upside down. Why? Because gravity is not strong enough to pull the thick oatmeal from the pot.

This is what happens when you don't drink enough water and end up dehydrated. When you don't drink enough water, you don't put enough water in your blood, causing your blood to become too thick. When the heart squeezes and pushes the thick blood up into the aorta, the blood has to fall down out of the aorta where the aorta bends. This is the equivalent of turning the pot of oatmeal upside down.

If the blood is too thick, gravity will not be strong enough to pull it down to your feet. Therefore, the muscles have to begin squeezing to push the blood down to your feet. Once these muscles squeeze, they increase the pressure inside the blood vessels, causing increased or high blood pressure. (http://www.optimumhealth.ws/Dehydration_High_Blood_Pres.html, accessed February 18, 2016)

Low blood pressure isn't necessarily unhealthy unless symptoms are present. Typical symptoms of low blood pressure from dehydration are dizziness, light-headedness, and fainting. Low blood pressure causes an inadequate amount of fluid to reach the organs, potentially causing strokes, heart attacks, or kidney failure and has causes in addition to that of dehydration. Low blood volume is a major contributor to low blood pressure; however, some medications and heart disease are also factors.

A friend of mine stopped by to say hello and chat about his most recent stubborn diagnosis of high blood pressure. He is in his seventies, a strong man with a military background, and he explained that he has always enjoyed good health, has taken vitamins religiously for decades, and eats healthy. His frustration was that his last several doctor visits had revealed high blood pressure, and during his most recent visit, his doctor said that if it didn't come down, he would definitely need to start taking blood pressure medication.

This advice was quite upsetting as my friend feels strongly about staying off all medications, if possible. I asked him if he keeps himself hydrated with water. He said, "No, I have really never been good about drinking water." Ironically, I was just finishing my research for this chapter and shared with him the importance of hydration and also explained about salts and mineral balance as well as pH balance. It sounded like a possible simple solution, and he said he would start right away. Two days later, he called me just to share his observations and the good news about his blood pressure with the addition of good hydration, adding a bottle of water with a pinch of Himalayan sea salt three times in the day. He said he was testing himself several times a day and had already dropped to numbers consistently in a healthier range. He was going to continue the regimen and was hopeful that it was the answer to his health dilemma. This is one of those real easy changes that really brings about noticeable positive results fast!

I have a fascinating story to tell in wrapping up this chapter, a story about Dr. Fereydoon Batmanghelidj, an Iranian-born, internationally known researcher and author who dedicated the last twenty years of his life to advocating the natural healing power of water. Dr. Batmanghelidj attended Fettes College in Scotland and graduated from Saint Mary's Hospital Medical School in London University, studying under Sir Alexander Fleming, who shared the Nobel Prize for the discovery of penicillin. In 1979, Dr. Batmanghelidj was held as a political prisoner during the Iranian Revolution and was in Evin Prison for almost three years. During that time, there were no medications available to him, so using the only resource available—water—he treated a fellow prisoner for a severe peptic ulcer. Within minutes of drinking two large glasses of water, the man's pain was gone. Dr. Batmanghelidj instructed him to drink two glasses every three hours. The man's pain went away and never returned. Dr. Batmanghelidj treated over three thousand fellow prisoners with water and conducted extensive research into the effects of preventing and treating different painful medical conditions with water. The doctor escaped from Iran and came to the United States in 1982, where he began his research on unintentional dehydration and its effects on the body. His findings were published in the *Journal of Science in Medicine Simplified* in 1991 and 1992. Here is what Dr. Batmanghelidj, discussing his treatments, said in his own words in an interview with the *Cincinnati Post*: "I truly am a missionary. And I have no commercial interest in selling water. I don't even tell people to go buy designer water. I have no ulterior motive other than truth." (WaterCure.com, accessed February 18, 2016)

Dr. Batmanghelidj wrote a popular and very informative book, *Your Body's Many Cries for Water: You are not sick; you are thirsty! Don't treat thirst with medications.* Many health practitioners agree with Dr. Batmanghelidj, believing that many illnesses can be reversed with the addition of good, consistent hydration. Here Dr. Batmanghelidj explains his findings and what he has deduced from them:

> Medications are palliatives. They are not designed or considered to cure the degenerative disease of the human body. The current practice of clinical medicine is based on the application of pharmacological chemistry to the human body. At the medical school, more than six hundred teaching hours are allocated to the use of pharmaceutical products. Only a few hours are allocated to instructions on diet and nutrition. The simple truth is that dehydration can cause diseases. Everyone knows that

water is good for the body, but that it is critical is for the most part overlooked.

We misinterpret thirst signals as pain, and treat them with drugs which silence instead of cure the problem. Because dehydration eventually causes loss of some functions, the various signals given by water distribution system regulators during severe and lasting dehydration have been translated as indicators of unknown disease conditions of the body. I discovered that histamine is a vital chemical messenger in the brain. Histamine has a most important function. It is in charge of water intake and drought management in the body. It is less active when the body is fully hydrated and becomes increasingly active when the body becomes dehydrated. To hush the body's call for water by masking the symptoms with drugs is like turning out the dashboard light that signals us that our car is about to overheat.

Every function inside the body is regulated by and depends on water. Water must be available to carry vital elements, oxygen, hormones, and chemical messages to all parts of the body. Without sufficient water to wet all parts equally, some more remote parts of the body will not receive the vital elements that water supplies. Without sufficient water to constantly wet all parts, your body's drought-management system kicks into action. The histamine-directed chemical messenger systems are activated to arrange a new, low quota of water for the drought-stricken area. If the dehydration persists and is not corrected naturally with water, it becomes symptom-producing and, in time, develops into a disease condition. (*Your Body's Many Cries for Water*, 1995)

His message may well be one of the most important health factors described in this book. This is one we can all use and experience instant rewards.

Chapter 12

SUPPORTING AN
AILING THYROID

This chapter wasn't in my original thoughts or outline when I started writing this book. However, in the background of my daily life, friend after friend was going to a doctor in the area for natural hormone therapy as a solution to their ongoing health problems, problems that were not being resolved through traditional medicine. Part of the initial workup and testing with this natural hormone doctor was to have blood work done and a thyroid test. It was amazing to me how wonderfully these friends responded to this therapy. The steady weight loss for most of them was encouraging enough, but they also got rid of their menopausal symptoms as well. The true proof of the fact that it really worked was that most of them had no insurance coverage for this alternative therapy but faithfully found the means to keep this therapy going as a regimental part of their daily personal-health program.

I realized that many of them had gone through quite a few incredibly stressful situations in their lives, and burnt-out adrenal function was a common denominator. Since I live in a small community, I knew their personal stories. The stories are not unusual in themselves in today's society, but living these stories is hugely debilitating to the individual having the negative life experience. Some of the stories I knew of were vicious divorces after long marriages, children with serious diseases, children with serious addiction issues, premature deaths of spouses or children, and crippling financial issues from job loss coupled with a downturn in the economy. My observation was a middle-aged population group with autoimmune disorders, hyperthyroidism or hypothyroidism, stubborn weight and blood-sugar issues, or even worse, a serious cancer, multiple sclerosis, fibromyalgia, lupus, or Lyme disease diagnosis.

I began to consider, *This is just a cross-section of the population. I wonder what this looks like on a larger population scale?* I started my research on the thyroid and found some good information to offer to help support and heal an ailing thyroid. This material can also build awareness for those trying to keep a healthy thyroid working properly. Just like the huge growing statistic of pre-diabetes and diabetes in the American population, thyroid disease has its own staggering statistic that continues to grow exponentially. Dr. David Brownstein, a family practitioner in conventional medicine, turned to holistic medicine to complement his specialized practice of treating thyroid disease. His conventional and holistic approach to thyroid conditions has made him an authority on the topic. He has written many books on the thyroid gland, and his extensive research provides the statistic that more than fifty-two million Americans have thyroid disorders that are linked to fifty-nine separate diseases, stemming from iodine deficiency and lack of important nutrients and minerals. (http://remodelingyourhealth.com/thyroid/, accessed February 18, 2016)

A huge segment of the population has symptoms but has gone undiagnosed. Dr. Brownstein believes that if an individual has many of the symptoms of a thyroid condition, but basic blood tests report that the thyroid is normal, the individual should press onward and insist on more extensive thyroid testing. The thyroid is a gland in the front base of the neck under the Adam's apple that wraps around the windpipe and is shaped like a butterfly. Its name is from a Greek adjective for "shield shaped." It's one of the largest endocrine glands, glands that secrete different kinds of hormones into the bloodstream. The thyroid produces two primary hormones, thyroxine (called T-4) and triiodothyronine (T-3), as well as another hormone of great importance called calcitonin. These hormones created by the thyroid play an important role in regulating the body's metabolism and calcium balance.

The most common problems with the thyroid are hypothyroidism, hyperthyroidism, and goiter. Common signs of thyroid problems are exhaustion and fatigue, inability to either gain or lose weight, swelling in the neck in the area of the thyroid, hair loss and dry skin, pain or aches without exertion, carpal tunnel and tendonitis, loss of sex drive, anxiety, panic attacks or depression, and constipation for an extended period of time. Hypothyroidism is underactive or low thyroid function, which means the thyroid does not produce enough of certain important hormones. Women, especially women over sixty, are more likely to be diagnosed with low thyroid. It can go undetected in the early stages—a time of just feeling tired and weak. However, if left untreated, it will lead to health problems, such as joint pain, infertility, obesity, and high cholesterol, which can lead to heart disease. The most common cause of hypothyroidism is Hashimoto's thyroiditis, which causes the body's immune system to attack the thyroid, causing the damaged gland to fail to produce enough thyroid hormones.

Symptoms of hypothyroidism occur slowly over time: tiredness, fatigue or depression, dry skin and brittle nails, intolerance to cold temperatures, memory problems or foggy thinking, irregular menstrual periods, and constipation. Chronic stress, mercury toxicity, and sources of chronic inflammation also lead to hypothyroidism. Chronic stress causes stress hormones that interfere with the function of the thyroid.

Mercury toxicity is most commonly found in dental fillings. Mercury and other heavy metals also interfere with normal hormone secretion of the thyroid. A growing major factor is autoimmune diseases from chronic inflammation. Chronic inflammation can lead to a multitude of inflammatory diseases, such as rheumatoid arthritis, psoriasis, osteoporosis, Alzheimer's, lupus, multiple sclerosis, fibromyalgia, polymyalgia rheumatica, colitis, Crohn's disease, diverticulitis, Parkinson's disease, heart disease, and cancer.

A source of chronic inflammation is the gluten found in wheat and other grains. There are many other foods that cause inflammation, such as harmful oils, artificial sweeteners and sugar, and food additives in processed and packaged foods. There are other foods to avoid as well when treating low thyroid function because they block the absorption of iodine, especially if these foods are raw. Cooking or roasting them reduces the negative effect on thyroid function. Here is a list of some of the foods that should be minimized to once or twice a week: almonds, broccoli, cauliflower, cabbage, kale, pears and peaches, turnips, Brussels sprouts, peanuts, spinach, soy, and pine nuts.

Foods that support and boost low thyroid function are also great sources of iodine. Some of these are listed below:

- Milk
- Cheese
- Eggs
- Yogurt
- Soy sauce (remember, gluten free)
- Saltwater fish
- Seaweed (nori, dulse, kelp, etc.)
- Shellfish

Meat and poultry are also inflammatory foods, so they should not be the main part of the meal. Following the alkaline foods chart in chapter 4 will help to eliminate chronic inflammation and support thyroid function.

Hypothyroidism is easily detected with a blood test. Upon starting treatment, relief of the symptoms is found in just a few weeks, with total recovery within a few months. A conscientious diet will prevent flare-ups and progression of disease.

The other end of the spectrum in thyroid function is hyperthyroidism. This is considered an overactive thyroid, when the thyroid overproduces hormones. Having too much thyroid hormone is also treatable, but without treatment it can lead to serious health problems. Common symptoms of an overactive thyroid are quick weight loss, sweatiness, fast heartbeat, nervousness, and moodiness. The major cause of most hyperthyroidism is Graves' disease, an autoimmune disease. Symptoms of Graves' disease come on gradually and include losing weight when eating more than usual; fine hair falling out; hot, sweaty skin that is red and itchy; shaky hands; fast heartbeat and breathing problems; more bowel movements than usual; bulging eyes; disturbed sleep; or feeling moody, weak, and tired.

The cause of hyperthyroidism can be from several sources. Noncancerous nodules in the thyroid, called nodular thyroid disease, are painless but can be felt when touching the location of the thyroid. These nodules stimulate an overactive response in the thyroid. Too much iodine also leads to an overactive thyroid. Certain heart medications contain a large amount of iodine, triggering hyperthyroidism; and sometimes, as a result of lack of follow-up or not following the correct dosage instructions, patients being treated for thyroid problems take an excessive amount of thyroid medication and cause the thyroid to become overactive.

There are foods to avoid when treating hyperthyroidism or Graves' disease. Understanding that the thyroid utilizes iodine to secrete hormones that balance metabolism and calcium and that hyperthyroidism is overactive glandular function, it makes sense to reduce foods that supply or help in the absorption of iodine. Avoid these foods or eat them sparingly:

- Processed foods (high sodium content)
- Iodized salt
- Sugar
- Caffeine
- Fried foods (if frying, use a friendlier oil, such as coconut or palm oil)
- Seaweed sources (kelp, nori, dulse, etc.)
- Red meat

Foods that minimize iodine absorption or block the thyroid from using iodine keep the thyroid from overproducing hormones. These foods are called goitrogens. Goitrogens can slow down the thyroid and naturally act as an antithyroid drug. Many of these foods are from the brassica family, or cabbage family: cabbage, broccoli, kale, cauliflower, turnips and rutabagas, Brussels sprouts, spinach, soybeans, and peanuts. Remember, eating these foods raw utilizes the enzyme that blocks the absorption of iodine much more than eating them cooked.

A third condition that can occur in the thyroid is goiter. Goiter is not cancer but is an enlarged thyroid gland. A goiter can be present with the thyroid function tests showing normal readings. This condition is not painful in itself, but it can cause swallowing problems and coughing disturbances. Goiters usually develop from the presence of a tumor or disease. Goiter is commonly caused by lack of iodine or low production of thyroid hormones, but it can also be present from an overactive thyroid and inflammation. Although goiters can be found in people of all ages, they are found mostly in women. A person with a goiter should eat a balanced diet, avoiding white flour and sugar products, fried or greasy foods, caffeine, flesh foods, and alcohol. A gluten-free (anti-inflammatory) diet of fresh organic or natural foods, with plenty of rest, exercise, fresh air, and water for good hydration, will provide a perfect platform to help resolve goiter issues. Inflammatory response is a condition of all thyroid disorders. At a minimum, all individuals should pursue a gluten-free diet to prevent further aggravation to the condition or any resulting diseases.

As I write this chapter, it becomes more and more obvious that all roads lead back to the same solution. Eating a diet that is alkaline; rich in minerals, vitamins, and nutrients; and free of any sources that lead to inflammation will go a long way in prevention and healing the body. Most people are driven to take action by the simple fact that they are frustrated with their weight, under or over, so they end up going to a doctor. This is when conditions like hypothyroidism are found as contributing factors.

I find it fascinating that other cultures with very large populations take an approach that is totally different from typical Western medicine. It's so relevant and important to be aware of other concepts and approaches available to restore and maintain overall health, especially serving the body's ability to maintain a healthy temperature.

In Eastern medicine, Ayurvedic holistic health began over five thousand years ago when Indian monks were looking for new ways to be healthy. The monks revered their bodies as temples and believed that preserving their health would allow them to develop more spiritually. In Ayurveda, food and lifestyle are the important medicines, and prevention is key. Body types, body temperature, alkalinity-acid balance, and metabolism are approached differently, but seemingly in a less complicated manner. Foods are considered cooling or warming in regard to what happens in the body once they are ingested. Body types, or *doshas*, are unique patterns of energy combinations of physical, emotional, and mental characteristics that make each individual a unique mix of three mind-body principles. The three doshas are *vata*, *pitta*, and *kapha*. Curious? Look below at these dosha descriptions and information:

Vata Dosha

Here are some of the common characteristics of people who have a predominantly vata constitution:

- Creativity, mental quickness
- Highly imaginative
- Quick to learn and grasp new knowledge, but also quick to forget
- Sexually easily excitable, but quickly satiated
- Slenderness; lightest of the three body types
- Talk and walk quickly
- Tendency toward cold hands and feet; discomfort in cold climates
- Excitable, lively, fun personality
- Changeable moods
- Irregular daily routine
- Variable appetite and digestive efficiency
- High energy in short bursts; tendency to tire easily and to overexert
- Full of joy and enthusiasm when in balance
- Respond to stress with fear, worry, and anxiety, especially when out of balance
- Tendency to act on impulse
- Often have racing, disjointed thoughts
- Generally, have dry skin and dry hair and don't perspire much
- Typical health problems include headaches, hypertension, dry coughs, sore throats, earaches, anxiety, irregular heart rhythms, muscle spasms, lower back pain, constipation, abdominal gas, diarrhea, nervous stomach, menstrual cramps, premature ejaculation and other sexual dysfunctions, and arthritis. Most neurological disorders are related to vata imbalance.

Physical Features of Vata Dosha

People of vata constitution are generally physically underdeveloped. Their chests are flat, and their veins and muscle tendons are visible. The complexion is brown, and the skin is cold, rough, dry, and cracked.

Vata people generally are either too tall or too short, with thin frames that reveal prominent joints and bone ends because of poor muscle development. The hair is curly and scanty, the eyelashes are thin, and the eyes lusterless. The eyes may be sunken, small, dry, and active. The nails are rough and brittle. The shape of the nose is bent and turned up. Physiologically, the appetite and digestion are variable. Vata people love sweet, sour, and salty tastes and like hot drinks. The production of urine is scanty, and the feces are dry, hard, and small in quantity. They have a tendency to perspire less than other constitutional types. Their sleep may be disturbed, and they will sleep less than the other types. Their hands and feet are often cold. Psychologically, they are characterized by a short memory but quick mental understanding. They will understand something immediately but will soon forget it. They have little willpower, tend toward mental instability, and possess little tolerance, confidence, or boldness. Their reasoning power is weak, and these people are nervous, fearful, and afflicted by much anxiety. Vata people tend to earn money quickly and also to spend it quickly.

Pitta Dosha

Here are some of the common characteristics of people who have a predominantly pitta constitution:

- Medium physique, strong, well built
- Sharp mind, good concentration powers
- Orderly, focused
- Assertive, self-confident, and entrepreneurial at their best; aggressive, demanding, and pushy when out of balance
- Competitive; enjoy challenges

- Passionate and romantic; sexually have more vigor and endurance than vatas, but less than kaphas
- Strong digestion, strong appetite; get irritated if they have to miss or wait for a meal
- Like to be in command
- When under stress, become irritated and angry
- Skin fair or reddish, often with freckles; sunburn easily
- Hair usually fine and straight, tending toward blond or red, typically turns gray early; tendency toward baldness or thinning hair
- Uncomfortable in sun or hot weather; heat makes them very tired and perspire a lot
- Others may find them stubborn, pushy, opinionated
- Good public speakers; also capable of sharp, sarcastic, cutting speech
- Generally, good management and leadership ability, but can become authoritarian
- Like to spend money and surround themselves with beautiful objects
- Subject to temper tantrums, impatience, and anger
- Typical physical problems include rashes or inflammations of the skin, acne, boils, skin cancer, ulcers, heartburn, acid stomach, hot sensations in the stomach or intestines, insomnia, bloodshot or burning eyes and other vision problems, anemia, and jaundice.

Physical Features of Pitta Dosha

These people are of medium height, slender, and their body frame may be delicate. Their chests are not as flat as those of vata people, and they show a medium prominence of veins and muscle tendons. The bones are not as prominent as in the vata individual. Muscle development is moderate. The pitta complexion may be coppery, yellowish, reddish, or fair. The skin is soft, warm, and less wrinkled than vata skin. The hair is thin, silky, red or brownish, and there is a tendency toward premature graying of hair and hair loss. The eyes may be gray, green, or copper brown and sharp; the eyeballs will be of medium prominence. The nails are soft. The shape of the nose is sharp, and the tip tends to be reddish.

Physiologically, these people have a strong metabolism and good digestion, resulting in strong appetites. The person of pitta constitution usually takes large quantities of food and liquid. Pitta types have a natural craving for sweet, bitter, and astringent tastes and enjoy cold drinks. Their sleep is of medium duration, but uninterrupted. They produce a large volume of urine, and the feces are yellowish, liquid, soft, and plentiful.

There is a tendency toward excessive perspiring. The body temperature may run slightly high, and hands and feet will tend to be warm. Pitta people do not tolerate sunlight, heat, or hard work well. Psychologically, pitta people have a good power of comprehension; they are very intelligent and sharp and tend to be good orators. They have emotional tendencies toward hate, anger, and jealousy. They are ambitious people who generally like to be leaders. Pitta people appreciate material prosperity, and they tend to be moderately well off financially. They enjoy exhibiting their wealth and luxurious possessions.

Kapha Dosha

Here are some of the common characteristics of people who have a predominantly kapha constitution:

- Easygoing, relaxed, slow paced
- Affectionate and loving
- Forgiving, compassionate, nonjudgmental nature; stable and reliable; faithful
- Physically strong with a sturdy, heavier build
- Have the most energy of all constitutions, but it is steady and enduring, not explosive
- Slow moving and graceful

- Slow speech, reflecting a deliberate thought process
- Slower to learn, but never forget; outstanding long-term memory
- Soft hair and skin; tendency to have large, "soft" eyes and a low, soft voice
- Tend toward being overweight; may also suffer from sluggish digestion
- Prone to heavy, oppressive depressions
- More self-sufficient; need less outward stimulation than do the other types; a mild, gentle, and essentially undemanding approach to life
- Sexually kaphas are the slowest to be aroused, but they also have the most endurance.
- Excellent health; strong resistance to disease
- Slow to anger; strive to maintain harmony and peace in their surroundings
- Not easily upset and can be a point of stability for others
- Tend to be possessive and hold on to things, people, money; good savers; don't like cold, damp weather
- Physical problems include colds and congestion; sinus headaches; respiratory problems, including asthma and wheezing; hay fever; allergies; and atherosclerosis (hardening of the arteries).

Physical Features of Kapha Dosha

People of kapha constitution have well-developed bodies. There is, however, a strong tendency for these individuals to carry excess weight. Their chests are expanded and broad. The veins and tendons of kapha people are not obvious because of their thick skin, and their muscle development is good. The bones are not prominent.

Their complexions are fair and bright. The skin is soft, lustrous, and oily; it is also cold and pale. The hair is thick, dark, soft, and wavy. The eyes are dense and black or blue; the white of the eye is generally very white, large, and attractive.

Physiologically, kapha people have regular appetites. As a result of slow digestion, they tend to consume less food. They crave pungent, bitter, and astringent foods. Stools are soft and may be pale in color; evacuation is slow. Their perspiration is moderate. Sleep is sound and prolonged. There is a strong vital capacity evidenced by good stamina, and kapha people are generally healthy, happy, and peaceful.

Psychologically, they tend to be tolerant, calm, forgiving, and loving; however, they also exhibit traits of greed, attachment, envy, and possessiveness. Their comprehension is slow but definite; once they understand something, that knowledge is retained. Kapha people tend to be wealthy. They earn money and are good at holding on to it. (http://www.holisticonline.com/ayurveda/ayv-basis-tri-dosha.htm, accessed February 18, 2016)

The site goes on to report that all individuals are a combination in some way of all three doshas, with one predominant. This is called *tridosha*, which means "healthy person." However, the proportion varies according to the individual, and usually one or two doshas predominate. Within each person, the doshas are continually interacting with one another and with the doshas in all of nature. This explains why people can have so much in common but can also have an endless variety of individual differences in the way they behave and respond to their environment.

Ayurveda recognizes that different foods, tastes, colors, and sounds affect the doshas in different ways. For example, very hot and pungent spices aggravate pitta, but cold, light foods such as salads calm it down. This ability to affect the doshas is the underlying basis for Ayurvedic practices and therapies.

A balance among the tridosha is necessary for health. Together, the tridosha govern all metabolic activities. When their actions in our mind-body constitution are balanced, we experience psychological and physical wellness. When they are somewhat unbalanced, we may feel uneasy. When they are more obviously unbalanced—when one or more of the three dosha influences is excessive or deficient—discernible symptoms of sickness can be observed and experienced.

In Ayurveda, foods are either cooling or warming. This is in alignment with the reaction they have on the body. Examples of cooling foods are avocados, cucumbers (hence, "cool as a cucumber"), green leafy vegetables, broccoli, zucchini, green beans, sweet potatoes, cherries, grapes, peaches, mangos, and pineapple. Summer is considered a pitta season, which requires cooling foods to be comfortable and balanced. Sweet, bitter, and astringent foods are best for cooling balance.

Examples of warming foods are tomatoes, onions, beets, spinach, garlic, curry, ginger, and cayenne. Dairy items such as cheese, sour cream, and yogurt are also warming foods. Winter is considered kapha season, calling for warm and spicy cooked foods with warming spices like cayenne, chili, cumin, ginger, and curries. Vata season is springtime, which includes a balance of fresh, raw cooling fruits and vegetables with a balance of warm, cooked foods and a balance of exercise and rest.

Traditional Chinese medicine practitioners use warming, cooling, and neutral foods (neither warm nor cold) to balance the body's yin and yang to treat disease. Yin means negative, dark, and feminine, and yang means positive, bright, and masculine. This said, listening to the body, regardless of vata, pitta, kapha, or yin-yang influences, should reveal your basic constitution, which represents your psychological and physical experience and nature. Achieving optimum health and healing starts with awareness and balance of all your environments: your thoughts, your diet, and your physical surroundings.

Chapter 13
MAINTAINING A HEALTHY WEIGHT

Maintaining a healthy weight can be just as frightening to the thin person who cannot gain a pound as it is for the overweight individual heading toward obesity. Either extreme can threaten an individual's quality of life. The reason I am writing this chapter on maintaining healthy weight is to address both ends of the health spectrum on the topic of weight. I believe it is information that is valuable and can be constructive knowledge to have at some critical point in life.

Huge weight loss during an illness or a treatment for an illness can be frightening and frustrating to the individual, his family, and friends. I remember when my daughter was initially sick, before her diagnosis, and she was home, too ill to go to school. I picked up her assignments at the middle school, and they gave me her school pictures with her homework. It was mid-October, and the school had taken the seventh grade's class pictures in mid-September. I opened them and burst into tears. She looked nothing like her healthy photos from a month earlier. She had already lost more than twenty pounds, and her hair, skin, and eyes were now ashen and dull. *Oh, my God*, I thought through the sobs, *what is happening to my dear daughter?* It was truly astonishing.

With her at home, trying to work through what we thought at the time was a bad virus, I hadn't noticed the dramatic change her body was going through. Yes, she was definitely sick and hadn't been out of bed much, but to see the pictures and realize how much she had lost in such a short period of time was horrifying. She had no appetite. She drank water and green tea for the most part and refused food because it made her nauseous. She was afraid eating would trigger dizziness and vomiting episodes. At the peak of her illness and hospitalization, she had lost seventy pounds from her initial doctor's visit with symptoms. It is amazing that she lost so much and is still with us today.

Emaciation or extreme weight loss is due to a loss of subcutaneous fat (the fatty, or adipose, tissue beneath the skin) and muscle throughout the body. Malnutrition and dehydration during hospitalization are treated with intravenous infusions, such as TPN (total parenteral nutrition), which is a drip run over a period of ten to twelve hours with a solution of carbohydrates, protein, fats, and electrolytes, or with a feeding tube or PEG line (percutaneous endoscopic gastrostomy) for a patient who cannot eat or should not eat during treatment and recovery.

Many patients are treated at home for disease and illness. Commonly, doctors recommend liquid nutritional products as home treatment for extreme weight loss and malnutrition. These products are over-the-counter or available in a grocery store. Most of these drinks have water, sugar, and corn syrup as the first and major ingredients. They also have carrageenan as a thickener, which can be inflammatory or disturbing to the digestive system. There are alternative, holistic nutritional supplement shakes and drinks that offer whole-food dietary supplementation and provide more nutrients, enzyme action, and pH balance for the recovering body. These products can be found in the natural-foods section of most large grocery stores, in health food stores, and online.

I would recommend staying away from sugar and corn-syrup-based products when treating any illness because of the body's inflammatory response to sugar. There are many products that are high in sugar, even though you won't see sugar as an ingredient on the package. Other words are often used that mean sugar but may be unfamiliar because they indicate the source of the sugar. Naturally occurring sugars can also be overconsumed by the unknowing patient or individual. Here are some of the most common: fructose, which is natural sugar from fruit; lactose, which is found in milk and dairy products made from milk, such as ice cream; and maltose, which is derived from grain. There is also glucose, which is a simple sugar found in plants; sucrose, which is made from glucose and fructose; and finally dextrose, which is a form of glucose.

The body requires glucose to feed the cells; however, it is best to get it from natural sources and in moderation. Natural sugars like honey, raw honey, maple syrup, molasses, agave nectar, monk fruit, and stevia provide nutrients and antioxidants in addition to the benefit of sweetening for taste and providing glucose for energy.

Glucose is absorbed directly into the bloodstream during digestion from simple or complex carbohydrates or sugars. Simple carbohydrates are absorbed very quickly into the bloodstream and can spike blood-sugar levels, which then quickly plummet, leaving the body feeling sluggish with low energy. Sugar and corn syrup are simple carbohydrates/sugars without much additional nutritional value; however, natural sugars are also simple carbohydrates/sugars that happen to have some nutritional properties. Complex carbohydrates are the better choice because they enter the bloodstream slowly, digest slowly, and leave the blood-sugar levels even or balanced. Complex carbohydrates/sugars are vegetables, whole grains (I always suggest gluten-free), brown rice, legumes, millet, and steel-cut or gluten-free oatmeal. The slow absorption and provision of steady nutrients and energy allows the body to recover healthy cells and rebuild the immune system.

When my daughter was sick, I realized it was best to offer her food like I had done when she was a toddler. Back then, if I gave her a plate with a lot of different kinds of food, she wouldn't eat any of it. The whole presentation of food on her plate, though I thought it looked healthy and balanced, made her feel overwhelmed. I learned quickly to give her tiny portions of one thing at a time. This always worked. I would start with her protein source in very small, bite-sized pieces; then I would add a few pieces of a vegetable and finally a starchy complex carbohydrate like rice, squash, or potatoes. Sometimes I had to provide them in separate small dishes. It wasn't a matter of right or wrong; it was just a matter of getting some good food into my busy child.

When I'm coaching a caregiver or a patient, I ask right away what state the patient is in for ingesting food and getting proper hydration. During an illness, there can be all different levels of eating challenges. They range from total inability to eat to ravenous states as a result of steroid medications. Of course, if swallowing is a problem, a feeding tube or intravenous fluid intake is the best choice, even at home. When starting with a feeding tube as the means of getting nutrition into the patient, it is important to get digestive enzymes into their system because the patient won't be chewing to infuse the necessary enzymes like amylase and lipase into the food. Real food can be utilized by building a base of necessary ingredients into a formula for the G-tube. This takes some patience and a bit of experimentation to get the right balance and consistency, but the proof is demonstrated in the improved energy and overall recovery of the patient. Working with a certified or registered dietician or holistic practitioner to get the right blend and balance for the diet is helpful and recommended.

Juicing is an excellent way to get enzymes into the diet from an array of raw vegetables and some fruits. Keep in mind the high sugar content of fruit and use more vegetables, and when using fruit, consider fresh lemon or lime juice for its alkaline properties once ingested or juiced berries for their low-sugar content and high antioxidant properties. Using a full-spectrum enzyme supplement by opening a capsule or two and putting it into the formula is also helpful in aiding digestion and absorption. The type of tradition of eating or diet the patient is accustomed to can be customized by choosing foods packed with nutrients.

Whether adhering to a meat, dairy, or plant-based diet, there are optimum foods to provide balance. Important nutritional elements can be attained by using meat broths or stocks. Simmer chicken and bones with vegetables in water; add herbs for digestion, such as ginger, dill, parsley, or cilantro; and include seaweed sources like kelp or nori for extra nutrients. Cooled and strained, the broth is a wonderful source of nutrition.

Essential oils, such as fish oil, olive oil, and coconut oil, can and should be added as well. These oils blend best if they are warm. In addition, vitamin and mineral powders or liquid supplements can be easily added to this liquid base. Raw milk, raw goat's milk, or raw eggs are also a good way to supply protein with enzyme content for easy digestion. Great products like hemp protein and whey are powerful sources of nutrition and protein for supplementing. Complete proteins from plant sources are quinoa, buckwheat, amaranth, spirulina, and hemp seed. In addition to being gluten free, these plant sources of protein are very nutritious and are good for fiber and energy. Quinoa (pronounced "kin' wa") is also a complete protein. Millet is also a very healthy grain, alkaline and easy to digest. It works well cooked, pureed, and strained to pump into a G-tube. Probiotics are very important for healthy digestion and elimination, and while they can be added from supplements, they are more convenient in the form of yogurt or kefir, a fermented dairy beverage, when trying to sustain a healthy liquid regimen.

All of this is important, but it can be quite a task to determine what works best for the preparer and the patient. Giving smaller infusions more frequently is usually tolerated better by someone who is extremely ill and weak. This also helps contribute to hydration. Keep the combinations simple and give infusions of food throughout the day; leave the night for fasting, allowing the body to detoxify and heal during sleep. All the elements of nutrition listed above are needed for the recovering patient who is still ingesting food on his own. It becomes really important to serve small portions more often and spread the different foods into smaller meals throughout the day.

Sipping on clear broth or stock, herb teas, and smoothies can balance nutritional needs, blood sugar, and aid hydration. Some days are better than others, but it is important to try various ways to get the most nutrition and hydration into the patient with the least amount of struggle. There are also holistic formula products, comprised solely of whole foods, on the market to provide this variety, and they can be ordered online if preparation from scratch is not always possible.

Steroids are often added to treatment protocols and can cause hunger to be sporadic. Consuming a variety of nutritious drinks or beverages throughout the day can take the edge off hunger, and eating six small meals instead of three large ones is healthier and more stable for the healing body. Again, it is important to leave the evenings for fasting, sleeping, healing, and restoring. If eating late is necessary, it's best to have a small snack of fruit or yogurt since they both will digest easily.

Gaining or keeping weight on is not always the problem; losing weight while trying to maintain or recover health can be just as daunting. Basically, the nutritional elements needed are the same: complex carbohydrates and protein, with as much from plants as possible to keep the body alkaline; essential fat from healthy oils; and enzymes and probiotics for assimilation and digestion. Hydration throughout the day can curb appetite and provide support for healthy nutrition.

In addition to good hydration, eating six small meals staggered throughout the day is better than spaced large meals to keep the metabolism higher and the blood sugar balanced; this pattern also helps avoid bouts of overwhelming hunger that can lead to cravings and destructive eating habits. Water-based soups and raw vegetables are great sources of nutrition and hydration and well tolerated, especially when eaten in small servings throughout the day. They are also filling and provide a lot of vitamins and nutrients with few calories. Herbs and spices can raise metabolism while providing great flavor, minerals, and antioxidants to the food.

Having a good enzyme and probiotic intake is extremely important, no matter the stage of healthy recovery. Maintaining stable blood sugar provides steady, even energy levels. Getting good hydration, vitamins, minerals, and good sleep is the added medicine we all need for restoration, healing, and overall maintenance of good health.

Chapter 14

SUPPORTING THE BODY
FOR CANCER RECOVERY

W hen there has been a new diagnosis, in the craziness of figuring out what to do about it, the stress and temporary lifestyle change can leave the patient and family feeling like sitting ducks. My thoughts quickly shift to what can be immediately done to change this state and empower everyone to work toward the direction of wellness for this individual.

I know from experience that feeling hopeless and helpless is a station of thought that you visit for a little while, but this station serves no purpose for anyone. There is plenty that can be done to move health in a positive direction. In my opinion, a focus on the positive actions available is the best place for the patient, family, and friends to put their energy. Making sure everything that goes into the body is positive, whether good, inspiring, loving thoughts or nutritious, healthy, supporting foods, is key.

Three all-consuming topics will possibly be turning over in the cancer patient's mind during this time. First is fear and the processing of those thoughts. The second area of concern is nutrition—what can and should be eaten? The third area of consideration is of medical protocol, surgery, or both. I truly believe that I have listed these in the order of importance.

Empowering the body to work at its peak performance while working through a cancer diagnosis is the best thing patients can do for themselves, their families, and their medical teams. If there is ever a time to get in top shape, it's now. Utilizing and supporting the body's ability to heal itself and focusing on what can be done to minimize side effects and quickly recover healthy cells are where the energy and focus need to be.

Any doctor will tell you that patients who are their own advocate or who have a good advocate, along with positive thoughts and attitude, can get through any protocol or procedure more easily and tend to recover more quickly. Also, taking a look at the daily diet and making changes in consideration of the healthiest choices goes a long way to support recovery. The behind-the-scenes work of good support from a caregiver, family, or friends, while keeping a positive outlook and optimum diet, also aid the medical team to serve the patient better and realize the best possible outcome for the patient's recovery.

This isn't just pleasant thought on my part. Remember earlier in the book we talked about stress and the physical effect it has on the body? This is real science, backed by real biochemical information about how thoughts can affect health. It's worth the time to address and work through a patient's fears and concerns. It's natural to avoid talking to someone about an illness and to simply pretend nothing has happened. Many patients do feel better, however, if you openly ask them about their type of diagnosis, what approach to treatment they are taking, and if they will need any help during that time.

It is comforting for them to be asked questions such as these: "Will you need a ride to and from treatment?"; "Is there someone to let your dog out?"; "Do you need meals prepared?"; "Is there someone to meet your children after school?"; or "Do you need a hand with housework?"

The answer probably will be no, most of the time, but just the fact that you asked will raise the spirits of the patient and will help them to feel supported and valued.

Supporting the body with the right foods is the next line of defense, but some things are more effective than others. Knowing that cancer feeds on sugar, cannot survive with oxygen, and if exposed to the immune system is immediately destroyed gives us some nutritional tools to work with. Here are a few weapons in our arsenal.

Ellagic acid is a natural phenol antioxidant found in many fruits and vegetables. Ellagic acid also breaks down the protective protein that a cancer cell uses to hide or cloak itself from being detected by the body's immune system. Foods with ellagic acid are common and easily incorporated into a daily eating regimen. Taking time to research plenty of foods with ellagic acid and how to incorporate them into a daily diet regimen is important. Here are some of the more common and popular ones: green tea, blueberries, blackberries, strawberries, grapefruit, lemons, oranges, apples, cherries, red grapes, red wine, kale, bok choy, maitake mushrooms, ginseng, turmeric, nutmeg, lavender, parsley, pumpkin, artichokes, tuna, tomatoes, olive oil, and dark chocolate with 70 percent cacao or more. As you can see, it will be easy to bring of few of these delicious choices into the front line of defense.

My studies and research have taught me that eating sugar and starches can lead to havoc in health. Sugar alone causes harm, but the body also converts simple starches to sugar for energy. This process can definitely be an added negative aspect in many illnesses and, if managed, can make all the difference in an individual's recovery. In general, illnesses improve more quickly and the body's ability to heal is more acute when simple sugars and starches are eliminated from the diet. This is especially so in a cancer diagnosis since cancer cells feed on sugar.

Just as it is important for a diabetic to control blood sugar, it is also very important for a cancer patient to get nutrition from foods that have a low glycemic or low sugar index. In the next chapter, I have provided a variety of food suggestions that have a low glycemic index.

This information is valuable for anyone for health maintenance but especially for those with cancer or blood sugar issues.

Eating alkaline foods and live foods for enzyme content is especially important to a cancer patient. Cancer does not grow in an alkaline environment but does in an acidic one. Cancer also is destroyed by oxygen and is weakened by hydration. Eating and drinking to support normal pH balance, digestion, and the immune system is not only essential, it is imperative.

Probably the easiest way to stop eating simple sugars and starches is to eliminate all packaged and processed foods. Eating a lot of fresh or frozen vegetables and some fruit supports a healthy pH balance. Going back to the basics and eating more simply will balance the diet without a lot of work. When natural-health coaches say to avoid the inner aisles at the grocery store and just shop the perimeter, it's because the refrigerated, fresh, whole foods are typically found on the outer edge of the store. Eating healthy foods raw or cooked very simply—without coatings, sauces, or gravies—allows the body to digest and process with more ease and to take full advantage of the nutrients and minerals present. And again, eating foods in a raw form eases the burden of the body by creating digestive enzymes to handle the intake.

If a patient is taking a treatment that causes the immune system to be compromised, the types of raw foods and how they are handled is important to control exposure to germs and bacteria. However, it is still important to get enzymes at this time—actually, it is critical—so taking a good-quality enzyme supplement with a variety of enzymes represented may indeed be the easiest and safest way to get through this time. Any work that is taken away from the pancreas and the body will support the recovery process.

Small, healthy, and balanced meals throughout the day are probably the best approach for the recovering cancer patient. On days that eating is very unappealing, drinking healthy smoothies may be the right answer. Preparing foods to be eaten in snack-style increments, rather than in big-meal format, also allows food to be readily available. Sometimes just the smell of something cooking is upsetting for the stomach of a cancer patient, making it difficult if not impossible to eat once the meal is ready.

It's optimum to eat raw and fresh and, if possible, local or organic fruits and vegetables, and if choosing to eat dairy and meat in the diet, it's optimum to use grass-fed or free-range organic sources as well. I know that this is not always an easy or affordable option for everyone, so the next best thing is to clean produce well after bringing it from the market before it's stored in the refrigerator.

For meats and dairy, look for sources that say no antibiotics or hormones used. No meats should be used that have nitrates in the ingredient list. Lunch meats, bacon, ham, pepperoni, hot dogs, kielbasa, etc., have preservatives called nitrates, nitrites, or sodium nitrate and sodium nitrites that are used in curing meats. These are synthetic preservatives that are unhealthy for the body. They have been linked to coronary, lymphatic malfunction cancer and other diseases and should always be avoided. Find the natural and organic meat section of the store. Companies can and do make these products without the harmful preservatives. Nitrates and nitrites are also in some commercial fertilizers, which have been proven as harmful to health, another reason organic food has grown in popularity. Again, make choices that have simple, real-food ingredients; ideally, the food that is being bought is the only ingredient on the package, or better yet, there is no package at all.

Cancer patients tend to crave sugar, so fruit will be the top choice as they move toward eating whole, natural foods. It is important to stick with small amounts of fruit at any given time, and it is best to eat berries since they have a lower glycemic index and boost immunity. Using products that are natural but harmless to blood-sugar levels, like stevia, or a low-glycemic alternative, like coconut sugar, will provide the sweet taste without any chemicals, artificial sweeteners, or simple sugars. Healthy choice sweeteners to be used in very small quantities are raw or local honey and 100 percent maple syrup.

Vegetables are typically the most essential food group and the most lacking in the typical diet. The phytonutrients, vitamins, and minerals from a variety of vegetables serve the body best and should be the first line of defense. Dr. Stone, our family doctor, said, "Eat from the outer perimeter of the grocery store and have the food on your plate look like a rainbow." Thinking about her words, I envisioned the nutrition and beauty of purple plums, grapes, and eggplant as well as blackberries, blueberries, limes, cucumbers, kale, spinach, kiwi, beets, raspberries, red apples, red peppers, oranges, squash, peaches, carrots, bananas, yellow peppers, and lemons. What a beautiful spread of wholesome nutrition—nice to visualize and even better to eat! Her advice applies to everyone—not just the sick, but the population in general.

Eating this way also supports an alkaline-acid-balanced diet. But don't consider it a diet, just think of it as good, balanced food choices that support the body to heal, recover, and maintain optimum health. My favorite alkaline foods are lemons, cucumbers, and avocados. I incorporate them into most of my meals in some way. Also, remember that fresh herbs are loaded with great nutrients and minerals and are alkaline and bring a lot of unique flavor to any dish.

We also need to discuss supplements. I believe in supplements when needed and have seen real results with patients who have worked to improve health by following good food choices and supporting the recovery of cells, organs, and the lymphatic and immune systems with herbal teas, mushroom and/or herbal complexes, aloe and sea-vegetable supplements, and antioxidants and immune-system boosters.

There is an herbal tea blend called Essiac tea, or it may be seen on the market as a "four-herb tea." *Essiac* is *Caisse* spelled backwards and is the name of the nurse from Canada, Rene Caisse, who saved many lives with her herbal formula tea, dating back to 1922. It feels therapeutic just making it. If you buy it in package form, it comes with each of the four herbs in an individual bag. You cook them together in a pot with water and follow the instructions to make the tea. When complete, drinking the tea hot or cold in portions as directed detoxifies the body and boosts the immune system. The original formula is burdock root, slippery elm inner bark, sheep sorrel, and Indian rhubarb root. The blend was modified later, adding watercress, blessed thistle, red clover, and kelp, and marketed as Flor Essence. There are other brands and modified formulas on the market that have similar properties. Any of them would certainly be helpful in detoxifying the body and boosting the immune system at some level.

When my daughter was finishing treatment for leukemia, she received a cancer-study protocol and was randomized to have interleukin-2 at the end of her treatments. I began studying everything about interleukin-2 since she was to receive it as an inpatient for two weeks after she was out of treatment. Try convincing a thirteen-year-old who has been in the hospital for nine months to go in for something else. There had to be a very good reason. To me, there was an enormous reason to go the extra step.

I had researched interleukin-2 and was so glad Monica could receive this treatment from her oncology team and was randomized to get it as part of her protocol. From all I had read, it was the synthetic version of mushroom therapy used in Eastern practices. The reason for adding this measure as the final step to Monica's protocol was to heighten the activity of her body's natural killer cells to seek out any leukemia cells that may have survived her treatments and destroy them. As I write this, I am realizing that was seventeen years ago this week, and Monica is alive and well and calling me right now on my cell phone. I again count my blessings.

Back to the mushrooms. While researching, I came across information about medicinal mushrooms used as supplements, which was very common in Eastern practices for treatments. Mushroom complexes are sold all over the world as nutritional supplements as well. The reishi, maitake, and shiitake mushrooms are the most common and are sold in proprietary blends by many companies. There are also other mushrooms with medicinal properties. There is a multitude of information about medicinal mushrooms and mushroom supplements on the Web.

A few years after Monica was out of treatment, I ran into one of my second cousins, waiting in a local law office that I do business with regularly for my real estate brokerage. We are from a very big family, so it's easy to lose track of each other. She was a beautiful, olive-skinned twenty-six-year-old, waiting her turn to see the attorney. I knew she had endured a bout with cancer of the salivary glands, which were removed, and I thought she was doing fine. As we sat together, she told me that her cancer had come back, and it was now in her lungs and liver. Her most recent doctor visits had indicated that her tumors were not responding to treatment and were too large for any cancer studies that were currently offered. She was told there was nothing else that could be done for her on the medical side and to get her things in order as her health would rapidly decline. She had made this appointment to write her will.

It was inconceivable; she looked better than some folks walking around with healthy doctor reports. I asked her if she was doing anything from a natural healing position, and she said she wasn't aware of anything she could do at that point. She told me she would be glad to do anything that would give her some hope. She wasn't ready to die, no matter how many arrangements she made to prepare. She wanted to experience falling in love, getting married, buying a home, and having a child. It didn't seem fair to be cut short of these wonderful experiences. She and I agreed to get together the next day and talk about some things I had learned in my research and while helping my daughter get through a terminal-cancer diagnosis.

We looked at what was available to her in natural healing and what made sense. She immediately started the alkaline-acid-based eating approach, following an alkaline-acid food chart similar to the one at the end of chapter 4. We also included Essiac tea (a tea blend that has its own interesting history and story), a combination of mushrooms in capsule form, and some liquid supplements for overall support with her vitamins and minerals. Equally important, we focused on keeping her elimination regular and detoxifying her body with all the natural ways we were aware of.

Just before she started eating alkaline, cleansing, and taking supportive supplements and antioxidants, one of her liver tumors was nine centimeters; there were several others that were smaller and many spots in her lungs. Within three months of eating alkaline and supporting all her body's natural functions, her largest tumor had shrunk to under five centimeters, which was the criterion for her to be eligible for an experimental treatment at a cancer center in Maryland.

Everything she was doing appeared to be slowing and reversing the cancer cells in her body. We were elated. The miracle of hope she had been praying for had arrived. She wanted to be eligible for a treatment, and now the opportunity was available.

Like Monica, my cousin continued her regular diet of alkaline-based foods during treatments and would just stop her vitamin and herb supplements during the immediate treatment phase. After the medicinal part of treatment became ineffective in her system, she would start again with a cleanse, a balanced alkaline diet, and vitamins and supplements to help detoxify, regenerate, and support her healthy cells.

After six years, cancer did return and sadly took this lovely young woman's life. She did have many wonderful personal successes during the extra time she had. She did find a great guy and married him; they bought a new home together and had a healthy son. She also taught us all valuable lessons of courage, determination, and kindness.

I present this story to provide some ideas and elements to be aware of. I am not suggesting that anything is a cure or a treatment. My hope is to expose everyone to alternatives I ran into on my quest to find information to promote healing and recovery of the body.

All the ideas here are meant to introduce more natural ways to support and recover health. I took a look at cancer recovery and will review diabetes next because both are so prevalent in our society. I want to offer as much information as possible to support the journey back to good health. Some of these alternatives stabilize and balance blood sugar in the body, which has a positive effect on managing diabetes, cancer, and hormonal issues—as well as aiding weight loss.

Chapter 15

GAINING CONTROL OF BLOOD-SUGAR LEVELS

A s a society, we have come to accept topics such as insulin resistance, low blood sugar (hypoglycemia), high blood sugar (hyperglycemia), pre-diabetes, and diabetes as common, ordinary illnesses that can affect anyone at any age. These ailments are so common, in fact, that when diagnosed, instead of having a reaction of instant fear and panic, patients are quite relieved that they can take a pill or give themselves insulin shots. In actuality, everyone should take a blood-sugar disorder as seriously as they would a cancer diagnosis.

In my life, I have witnessed how this illness, seemingly unthreatening in the beginning, is a very tough disease to get under control and heal if not taken seriously. My mother-in-law and a close personal friend had type 2 diabetes—*had* being the key word. They are no longer with us as they succumbed to the illness after many years of trying to control their blood sugar with insulin and diabetes medications.

In both cases, their diet was always in question. My sweet mother-in-law could never accept that the things she loved most in life could kill her. She loved funnel cakes at the local fairs, pancakes with syrup, and butter-pecan ice cream; she prided herself on baking the best cookies, brownies, and cakes. There was never a meal served in her home that didn't come with dessert.

A very close friend and his wife were twenty years younger than my mother-in-law, but both passed away in their sixties from complications of diabetes. Although both eventually passed from strokes, our dear friend suffered for years prior with circulation and diabetes complications that caused him to lose his toes and, later, both of his feet through amputation. They struggled with what to eat and mostly enjoyed sweets, fruits, and carbohydrate-heavy meals. It was difficult for them to break the cycle of eating the way they were accustomed to.

As a guide, normal blood-glucose or blood-sugar levels are in a range of 80–120 milligrams per deciliter (mg/dL), although this range can vary from lab to lab. So let's take a look at the variation of symptoms, conditions, reactions, and diseases that describe blood-glucose levels that are not normal, such as hypoglycemic, hyperglycemic, insulin resistant, pre-diabetic, and diabetic.

Hypoglycemia is a low blood-glucose or low blood-sugar condition or reaction characterized by blood-glucose (blood-sugar) levels usually less than 70 mg/dL and can occur in people with or without diabetes. Hypoglycemia is often a medical emergency that arises from an inadequate supply of glucose, the body's main energy source, to the brain. Some symptoms of hypoglycemia are sweating, extreme hunger, shakiness and feeling weak, dizziness, blurry vision, headache, and anxiety. More dramatic symptoms in a progressed state might be irritability and confusion, lack of stability to walk or stand, slurred speech, extreme emotions, and an inability to focus or concentrate. Very severe symptoms are coma, seizure, stroke, or even death.

I had a woman in her mid-fifties contact me through a friend. She said she was waking in the night with anxiety, and by morning she would awaken in a full-blown panic attack. She explained that she had undergone a hysterectomy four years earlier, so she was sure it wasn't hormone related. To her, it really seemed more like anxiety. We discussed her diet, sleep patterns, and elimination habits, and we discovered together that she ate very little protein or fat and had totally eliminated all salts. Her daily intake included mostly carbohydrates, with marginal hydration.

First, we experimented. I had her make a combination with almond butter, cinnamon, and a few other ingredients that I call my "blood stabilizer recipe." You can find it at the end of the book. This is a delicious combination of balanced nutrients. My thought process was if it was low blood sugar and she was eating mostly carbohydrates, these foods would convert to sugar and send her blood-glucose level high. When her blood sugar dropped, it would have no protein or fat to slow down the absorption of the sugar into the bloodstream so it could be properly metabolized. This rapid blood-sugar drop would leave the body shaky and weak, ultimately making her wake up in a state of panic. Many individuals wake up sweaty and/or panicked when their blood sugar is not stable. Insulin is a hormone, and it can certainly bring on an anxiety attack for anyone with too many carbohydrates and not enough protein and healthy fats in his diet.

The recipe I suggested she make would give her fats, protein, and a bit of carbohydrates with healthy salt and trace minerals for assimilation. Utilizing the findings I explained in chapter 7, "Finding Cures with Coconut," that coconut would enter the bloodstream without the need of normal digestion to be absorbed. Coconut oil starts being absorbed while still in the mouth and takes other nutrients with it. This is why the recipe requires the addition of a bit of coconut oil, and should not be replaced by an alternative oil. This action to reverse her low blood sugar would be immediate. I told her to eat some of the almond butter concoction, possibly a tablespoon, before going to bed to see how it affected her.

The first morning after, she called me amazed and excited. She had taken only one teaspoon of the almond butter recipe on a cracker before going to sleep. I had forgotten to tell her no crackers and to eat just the almond-butter mixture. She reported that she woke up after a much longer-than-usual period of sleep to some weak shakiness and a bit of anxiety, so she immediately took a second teaspoon of the mixture, chewing and swishing it in her mouth a bit before swallowing. To her amazement, in a few seconds the feeling totally subsided and went away. It was like a switch turned the feeling off. We had found the right answer for her. We started looking at different protein and fat sources she could add to her diet and also some proper things for her to eat before bed.

This woman loved eggs and egg salad, which she had long ago given up. She carried the common fear of high cholesterol and high blood pressure, two conditions she had previously struggled with and had never been able to reduce or eliminate, even though she gave up eggs, fats, and salt. The old dogma that eggs are bad for you has been wonderfully corrected in recent years to reveal the truth that eggs are really good in the diet. The body also needs healthy fats and salts to function properly. I suggested she eat a hard-boiled egg or egg salad before bed and have the almond-butter mixture by her bedside just in case she woke up with low blood sugar. It was a successful program for her, and now she is incorporating good salt with trace minerals, good hydration, and healthy fat and protein sources in each meal to keep her blood pressure, blood-sugar level, and cholesterol level balanced and in a healthy range.

Hyperglycemia is high blood glucose, or high blood sugar. This condition is realized when an individual has a consistent range of blood glucose above 126 mg/dL. This range is from the American Diabetes Association guidelines. This is the part that is really frustrating to me. There are often no symptoms early on, but when blood-glucose levels stay above normal for years, very serious complications arise.

An individual becomes insulin resistant, and his condition progresses to pre-diabetes or, even more progressed, diabetes. It really seems like the disease comes on almost overnight, when in fact it has been brewing in the background for years.

In my more elementary thinking, I have often wished that our bodies would just freeze, stop, and let us know when things are going on in our bodies that are wreaking havoc so there would be absolutely no choice but to immediately take corrective actions. My father was a mechanic, and he made sure we knew how important it was to service our vehicles so they wouldn't break down. An occasional bad battery, flat tire, or empty gas tank would leave us stranded. Our bodies don't come equipped with bright warning lights, and unlike our vehicles, we are self-repairing. Our bodies are miraculously forgiving, so we fail to get the big messages as quickly as we do with our vehicles.

When we eat, the stomach breaks food down into sugars, such as glucose, which is the main source of energy for the body. When glucose enters the bloodstream, the blood-sugar level begins to rise. The rise in blood sugar sends a signal to the pancreas to make insulin, a protein hormone produced by the body in the pancreas to metabolize (convert to energy) carbohydrates, sugars, and fats. The pancreas releases insulin into the bloodstream, where the insulin acts as a chaperone to take glucose into the cells for energy.

Each cell in the body has receptors. When the cell's receptors respond that there is enough glucose in the cells, insulin is no longer able to bring glucose into the cells. However, in the case of high blood sugar, the cells won't take more glucose/sugar, even though there is still plenty in the blood. The insulin cannot perform its normal function. Eventually the beta cells in the pancreas increase their production of insulin, trying to adjust for the lack of insulin going into the cells. But the cells have become resistant to taking insulin and using it effectively. This leads to hyperglycemia. Eventually the pancreas can no longer keep up with the demand for insulin, and excess glucose is still left in the bloodstream, leading to type 2 diabetes.

Type 2 diabetes is chronically high blood-glucose/sugar levels. Treatment usually requires changing the diet and taking metformin or insulin, depending on the stage of the diagnosis. Metformin is sold as Glucophage and is an anti-diabetic drug. It is prescribed when there is still normal kidney function. Metformin suppresses glucose production by the liver. There are some common side effects of metformin: diarrhea, decreased appetite, stomach discomfort, hoarseness or cough, lower back pain, muscle cramping, painful urination, and sleepiness. Less common side effects include anxiety, blurred vision, confusion, depression, sweats, headache, nightmares, shakiness, shortness of breath, and wheezing.

A percentage of patients taking metformin experience a medical emergency of lactic acidosis. Signs of this are vomiting, abdominal pain, nausea, dyspnea, hypothermia, and hypotension. Metformin can also cause a malabsorption of vitamin B-12. Subnormal vitamin B-12 levels can result in anemia or neuropathy. Supplementing with a B-100 or B-complex vitamin or B-12 shots may be necessary to support better blood-cell production and restore the patient's energy and stamina.

Human insulin is a peptide hormone and is central to regulating fat and carbohydrate metabolism in the body. Synthetic insulin was made from a combination of chemicals between 1966 and 1975. In 1978, scientists from Genentech cloned the human gene for insulin and placed it in *E. coli* bacteria. They grew large quantities of this bacterium, which started producing human insulin. They harvested the bacteria and purified the insulin. Clinical trials showed that the new insulin was effective in controlling diabetes. Genentech licensed the process to make this insulin to Eli Lilly. Eli Lilly has produced it since 1982. The main medical approach to controlling the progression of diabetes since that time has been the use of injected insulin.

Insulin resistance is also known as syndrome X, or metabolic syndrome. It is also considered pre-diabetes. Perimenopausal women experience a higher-than-average diagnosis of insulin resistance. Insulin is a major hormone, and if it is out of balance, minor hormones such as estrogen, progesterone, and testosterone will be out of balance as well. If hot flashes are present, so is insulin resistance, and it is impossible to get past hot flashes if insulin resistance is not addressed first.

In an article by OB/GYN nurse practitioner Marcelle Pick, from the website *Women to Women*, we read the following:

Over 80 million Americans suffer from insulin resistance, and it appears to sit at the center of a web of related health problems. Women who are insulin resistant are at much greater risk of obesity, diabetes, hypertension (high blood pressure), heart disease, high cholesterol, breast cancer, and polycystic ovarian syndrome (PCOS). There is some evidence that insulin resistance may contribute to endometrial cancer. It has also been implicated in Alzheimer's disease. Insulin resistance often accompanies the most common complaints we hear at *Women to Women*—fatigue and weight gain. As women approach menopause, they become increasingly intolerant of carbohydrates and find it easier to gain weight, especially around their waists. Afternoon blahs, sugar crashes, and carbohydrate cravings may all be early insulin resistance symptoms. (https://www.womentowomen.com/insulin-resistance/what-is-insulin-resistance/, accessed February 18, 2016)

I have explained why we need to get blood sugar under control, so next let's look at how to approach controlling blood sugar. The exciting thing I have learned from researching this topic inside and out is that it can be stabilized, reversed, and even eliminated. I have even read statements from holistic practitioners who teach alkaline healing and balanced nutrition who have not only reversed type 2 diabetes, but also witnessed type 1 diabetes stabilize and be controlled with this approach.

The body will respond right away to a good diet regimen that stabilizes hormone secretions and blood sugar. It will start to reflect balance and harmony with hormone and enzyme production. A proper diet that stabilizes blood sugar is truly the best diet for everyone. Learning about foods and their glycemic index is imperative to support the body and the metabolism of glucose/sugar.

The advice for middle-aged women with hypoglycemic symptoms, levels below 70 mg/dl, can also help with hyperglycemia, pre-diabetes, and diabetes. If an individual eats fewer foods that contain sugar and fewer carbohydrates/starches that convert to sugar and eats a balance of good fats and protein with each meal or snack, the food is absorbed slowly and the sugar level will stay steady, allowing the body to utilize and metabolize the food without swings in the blood-sugar level. Good hydration in between meals is also very important in metabolizing and utilizing food.

Getting familiar with a glycemic index as a useful tool to guide your diet away from foods too high in sugar content or sugar conversion is extremely helpful. The glycemic index is a measurement of carbohydrate-containing foods and how quickly blood-glucose/sugar levels rise after eating a particular food. A glycemic index chart   shows a food source and corresponding number index, revealing low-, medium-, or high-sugar impact on blood-sugar levels.

Choosing low-glycemic foods; eating plenty of vegetables that provide essential minerals, vitamins, nutrients, and antioxidants; and adding healthy fats and protein sources on a consistent basis will lead the body to healing itself, reduce body weight, bring blood sugar into a proper range, and bring blood pressure and alkaline-acid levels to normal pH balance. The need for intervention with pharmaceutical medications will decline as these levels, monitored by a physician, start to come to optimum levels.

Here is a condensed list of healthy food choices that are low glycemic/low sugar with high nutritional value that should be **increased** in the diet with a glycemic index below fifty-five: artichoke, broccoli, celery, cherries, cucumber, eggplant, grapefruit, green beans, lettuce (all varieties), peach, peppers, plum, snow peas, spinach (best cooked), summer squash, sweet potato, and tomatoes.

Here is a list of poor-quality, empty-calorie food choices to **avoid** that are also considered low glycemic/low sugar: pound cake, potato chips, ice cream, milk chocolate bars, and candy bars with peanuts.

Further, it is important to know examples of high-glycemic/high-sugar foods to **avoid** that have a glycemic index above seventy: rice cakes, bagels, most commercial cereals, cookies, most breads and rolls, corn chips, baked potato and instant mashed potato, kaiser rolls, doughnuts, frozen waffles, French fries, and pretzels.

The best way to quickly stabilize blood sugar that is very unstable is to eliminate sugar and grains completely and rely on vegetables, berries, lemons and limes for the carbohydrate component of your menu. The results are amazing. One week of this approach along with good hydration can improve energy levels immensely; doing it for thirty days is life changing!

Taking an active role in supporting the body's biochemical process includes balancing the diet with food choices that keep the blood sugar stable throughout the day. This eliminates the lows that cause bouts of tiredness or fatigue shortly after eating a meal. Taking diligent steps to stabilize blood sugar is a bold move toward reversing aging and illness. Recovery of energy and vitality is observed very quickly when processed foods are eliminated and quality nutrition becomes the norm.

Chapter 16

CHANGING THE VIBRATIONAL ENERGY OF THE BODY

This chapter has actually been the most fun for me to research, experiment with, and share. Early on in my quest to understand how the body works and how it heals itself, I learned about the vibrational frequency that exists in all matter and its significance in the body. The first person to develop the idea of healing with radio frequency was Albert Abrams, MD (1864–1924), who developed thirteen different devices to treat diseases by applying different frequencies. It was then developed further by Dr. Rife. In the late 1920s, Dr. Royal Raymond Rife, a medical doctor, developed a frequency generator. My interest in the story of Rife was that he claimed to successfully treat people with incurable cancer with his frequency generator. According to Rife, every disease has a frequency. He found that certain frequencies could prevent disease and others could destroy disease. He also discovered that substances that had a higher frequency could destroy the diseases of a lower frequency. There is a great website created to preserve the work and stories of the life of Dr. Rife at http://rife.org/.

Others believed in his work and were on similar paths of discovery and healing. American inventor Nikola Tesla (1856–1943), a pioneer of electrical technology, said that if we could eliminate certain outside frequencies that interfered in our bodies, we would have greater resistance to disease. Likewise, Dr. Robert O. Becker, in his book *The Body Electric*, also explained that a person's health can be determined by the frequency of the person's body. Today you can Google "vibrational frequency of___," and anything you can think of (sleep, peace, focus, concentration, etc.) will come up to be researched and explained. Use frequencies to get better sleep, reduce stress, stimulate the thyroid, stimulate hormones, improve clarity of thinking, bring peace and relaxation, experience abundance and prosperity, etc.

About a decade ago, I was presenting a series of health-recovery workshops with Denise Abda, who also coaches individuals with illnesses and disease. We showed slides of colored pictures of all different foods people might eat and the energy in hertz reflected in the food. The pictures were taken with a special light that showed different frequencies in color. We had some with vegetables and a red lentil that had high, colorful sparks rising from it and one of a cheeseburger on a bun that had a whitish glow above it with no spark or color range. It was all very interesting and a great way to illustrate how food gives us a corresponding energy spark or not.

At the time, Denise had purchased a Rife machine called the Detox Box. We followed the manual and had people set a frequency, based on their illness. It actually provided a frequency higher than the illness in order to create a frequency to reverse the disease and at the same time aid in detoxifying the body. I ended up purchasing one and have used it through the years as another tool in my bag of endless possibilities to create an avenue for healing. I can't say that I saw the results claimed by Dr. Rife, but the boxes, in all fairness, never left our offices and were just used randomly by people, not continually or consistently.

With that being said, here is a little observation I did have. A friend of mine was staying with me for months because her home had flooded and she had tried to repair it herself. Her exposure to black mold created a horrible health situation for her that affected her lungs and left her weak. She took many courses of antibiotics over a six-month span. She began to try holistic eating and other modalities as she feared she would never recover. Eventually she tried my Detox Box with the crystal hand rods. Every morning I would find her at my dining room table with it, running a breathing and lung-disease program. She insisted it was the only thing that gave her relief.

Within a few weeks of using the box religiously, she began to regain her strength and got her immune system back in working order. Eventually she overcame her illness. The Rife machine has been improved over the years and is still sold. Other companies have also developed products using this technology, but they are not as popular as some easier approaches that have been offered to the public for free. Personally, I find that people get more enjoyment by using a set of headphones and listening to isochronic tones and binaural beats from their computer, iPad, or smartphone to experience frequency therapy. One can go to YouTube and type in "isochronic tones and binaural beats for sleep" and get a huge variety of recordings to listen to, from five minutes of recording to eight-hour recordings. There are literally thousands of frequency videos to listen to on YouTube to treat anything you can think of. There are binaural beats for sleep and binaural beats for peace, meditation, and relaxation, etc.

The human brain produces different levels of electrical activity, depending on the amount of information it is processing. During a detailed task, it lights up with electrical charges as it sends and receives messages at a high concentration, its neurons firing in quick succession. While in a relaxed state of sleep, it glows more dimly, its neurons firing less often. This brain-wave activity is calculated by electroencephalographs (EEGs), machines that gather data from electrodes adhered to the skull to measure the frequency (the amount of electric activity per unit of time) in hertz. Measurements of electrical activity in the brain are more commonly referred to as brain waves. Some examples of brain-wave patterns are listed below:

- Gamma (25–100 Hz): most apparent at 40 Hz: heightened sense of consciousness, bliss, and intellectual acuity subsequent to meditation
- Beta (12–30 Hz): the normal, awake consciousness associated with busy tasks
- Alpha (8–12 Hz): the relaxed and reflective state, like that induced by closing the eyes during waking hours
- Theta (4–7 Hz): a very relaxed state associated with meditation and some sleep states
- Delta (3 and under Hz): deep, dreamless sleep

Gamma waves have been observed in Tibetan Buddhist monks, giving thought to the possibility of correlation between transcendental states and gamma waves. Theta waves are the sweet spot for many brain functions, providing the experience of extreme relaxation, creativity, and vibrant mental imagery. Throughout the day, the brain waves move between the latter four types of brain-wave patterns. Scientists and science-minded individuals with curiosity about brain-wave patterns have developed various audio techniques to induce different brain waves on demand. Many find these techniques an interesting psychological science to experience. I personally listen to binaural beats and/or isochronic tones for relaxation and meditation. I have enjoyed a variety of free recordings sampled from YouTube and others I have purchased.

Binaural auditory tones are auditory-processing artifacts, or apparent sounds, caused by specific physical stimuli. This effect was discovered in 1839 by Heinrich Wilhelm Dove and earned greater public awareness in the late twentieth century based on claims coming from the alternative medicine community that binaural beats could help induce relaxation, meditation, creativity, and other desirable mental states. The effect on brain waves depends on the difference in frequencies of each tone: for example, if 300 Hz was played in one ear and 310 in the other, then the binaural beat would have a frequency differential of 10 Hz.

This binaural-beat-frequency differential actually produces a phenomenon in the brain in which the difference between the left-ear and right-ear tones is heard in the brain as a third distinct tone or beat. This tone interpretation by the brain is a unique tone to each individual as the brain actually is creating a third tone as it tries to interpret the other two tones.

Are beats and tones for everyone? Definitely not. It's my intention to build awareness of this popular concept, but I must also inform you that there are health and safety-related warnings throughout any information you find about beats and tones that implore users not to listen to beats or tones while operating machinery or a motor vehicle. If one suffers from a medical condition, has a pacemaker, is pregnant, has had epilepsy or a mental illness, etc., consulting a doctor is highly recommended as a doctor should be able to determine whether the condition is severe enough that beats and tones would have an adverse effect. So I believe these statements are important and given for good reason in almost all product-promotion materials for binaural beats, monaural beats, and isochronic tones.

However, this concept has gained popularity; it's truly incredible how much information there is on the topic. I have been fascinated by the idea that having a different tone coming into each ear actually creates a tone that is unique to every individual as it's based on his brain's perception of the tones. Though it sounds complicated and crazy, it works for many. All you really need is a good set of headphones and you can listen to literally thousands of different direct healing topics. It's all auditory information, so CDs or Internet downloads are typically the sources for the content.

There are two other tones that I mentioned, which you will find while searching different beats and tones. One is isochronic tones, and the other is monaural tones. Isochronic tones are regular beats of a single tone used for brain-wave entrainment. Similar to monaural beats, the interference pattern that produces the beat is outside the brain, so headphones are not required for entrainment to be effective. Isochronic tones are a newer technology of brain-wave entrainment than monaural and binaural beats, and isochronic tones may be considered a more effective approach to brain-wave entrainment.

I found helpful information at www.project-meditation.org concerning the beats and tones. This site explains that monaural beats are produced when two tones combine digitally or naturally before the sounds reach the ears as opposed to combining in the brain like binaural beats and that monaural beats and isochronic tones have an advantage because you can listen to them without headphones. The site also asserts that many people who do not respond well to binaural beats often respond very well to isochronic tones.

All this information caused me to look at my body's energy differently. I started using my feelings like a GPS. Does this information, offer, person, building, town, meeting, question, or experience leave me feeling better or worse? When I truly started paying attention to how I was wired and how the vibration of all things or people I encountered either left me feeling good, lighter, peaceful, and joyful or, on the other hand, feeling bad, heavy, anxious, nervous, sad, angry, or exhausted, I immediately started changing my overall life experience. I have made more satisfying choices of how to spend my time, energy, and even money. Becoming more aware of other people's energy, whether positive or negative, gave me contrast and helped me realize better choices overall.

Using the body's natural GPS of thoughts and emotions to navigate to a better health experience, whether it is physical or mental health, requires staying in the moment and making each choice the best possible choice in that moment—even if that choice is to make no choice. This creates an immediate positive change for the body's vibrational energy and offers another method of feeling better.

Chapter 17
OVERCOMING OBSTACLES

T he day of any diagnosis is a big, somewhat crippling day for the body. It's the day that a sickness or pain is labeled with a name. Sometimes people spend weeks, months, or even years not really feeling up to par before they begin the journey of potential self-diagnosis. They may read magazines that scantily outline symptoms of an illness or go online and research all the possible diseases and conditions that have similar symptoms. All this information may leave them more frightened than before and without any resolution. Eventually they may end up in a doctor's office for tests, scans, scopes, and possibly biopsies to uncover the mystery of the illness or pain.

This journey of realizing something in the body is not right to the day of actual diagnosis is a time of worry, anxiety, and suffering, without much, if any, healing taking place. Actually, the opposite happens: things continually get worse. Most diagnoses carry a concrete public opinion about what happens to an individual once diagnosed with a particular illness or disease. Along with that, the doctor or medical team usually provides a projected typical progression of an illness. This takes the worry or fear, validates it, and sends it on a journey predicting the outcome. Sometimes the news is good or okay, but many times it's not.

In an instant, the conscious and subconscious loss of hope that takes place during negative news is very debilitating. This can create a negative path for the body and mind to follow. My message here is this: don't take this journey. Refuse to think that the outcome is the same for everyone. Refuse to think that recovery is not a possibility. Refuse to accept information that doesn't sound right. Expand the possibilities for recovery; expand the research; expand and gather more points of view and options. Use them all—or at least what makes sense—and get to a better place. From there, make the best, informed choices possible.

I totally believe in and have witnessed miraculous recoveries. There is a plethora of stories throughout the centuries of miraculous recoveries. They can be anyone's story if he is not defeated by the message of the diagnosis. When my daughter was hospitalized, especially at the time of her diagnosis, I refused to let anyone into her room without preparing him for what he would see and telling him how I expected him to handle it. If he didn't think he could do it, he didn't come in. I explained her current condition, what she looked like, and what the medical team was currently working on or concerned about, but then insisted that the visitor look at her with supporting, loving eyes and joke around with her and be light. In other words, I insisted he act like he always had around her and feel happy for her. I wanted each visitor to send the message that she would get well, that she was loved and supported and in good hands. Anything short of that absolutely could not come into her room. It took a while before all our family and friends could overcome their fear and come and visit her with positive expectations, but eventually they all came around.

I admit it sounds extreme and unusual, but I had a choice to make, and my daughter was twelve years old, sensitive, emotional, and searching for information in the faces of everyone who came into her room. She wondered if she looked horrible; she wondered if the doctors looked concerned because she was getting worse; and she wondered if the fear of others meant that we should have more fear. What was the message being given with their expressions?

So my action was to insist that everyone give her hope, love, support, and a good ribbing because she enjoyed the healthy sport of joking and sarcasm. Being proactive to set the bar for the most positive experience in every moment became my focus every day during the year of her hospitalization. We didn't wait for her hair to sadly fall out slowly, clump by clump. Her friends came, had a party with her, and took turns shaving her head over the side of her hospital bed. Then they gave her a pile of gifts that represented the coolest of caps and hats on the market. We were kind and lighthearted with the hospital staff and didn't probe the doctors about what would happen next. We had chosen them, and we believed in our choice. We knew it was the best choice for us. We asked questions—lots of questions—when things didn't make sense and reviewed new and better options when they presented themselves. We tried to find something that brought normalcy to each moment, like giving her medical team her favorite music CD to play when she was going in for a procedure or simply lying in bed together, watching a good movie or a favorite sitcom just like we did at home.

When all her treatments were finally over and she was considered by her doctors to be in remission, we went home. She was weak, thin, pale, and bald. The day we got home, I called the moms of all her friends and invited them to come over with their kids the next day for lunch. The new school year was about to start, and I needed to pave the way for her to have a support team of friends who knew the truth about her disease, her treatment, and what she needed to get through the day. It was actually a great day. It started out with a bit of uncertainty as I watched Monica on and off the couch throughout the morning, fussing with her clothes and hats, trying to make sure she looked her best and as cool as possible.

Then they arrived. One by one they came in and jumped onto the couch, hugged her and each other, teased each other, and rolled around in laughter. Once they were all there piled and cuddled around her, she spontaneously ripped her hat off; there was a moment of silence, then a huge burst of laughter. *She's back*, I thought as I settled in to catch up with the other mothers.

As everyone left that day, they were fully informed about Monica's illness, her treatments, and what her friends could do to help her. They all had many questions and concerns, such as "Can she drink from our water bottles?" and "Is leukemia contagious?" What a perfect setting to teach them, release their fears, and provide the next natural step for healing for Monica. She didn't have to worry about what was next; she was back with her friends, and they would protect her and pave the way for her to fit back into the life she had been away from for a year.

Many times, obstacles are what we think and make of them. As the saying goes, "Don't get ahead of yourself." Stay in the moment. By changing the approach to an illness to a positive, proactive flow of what to do next in each circumstance, moment, hour, day, etc., one brings the best possibility for good and continual progression to wellness.

Finding the right path for healing is definitely different for every individual. Suggesting many possibilities and potential tools that are within everyone's grasp in order to recover and maintain good health was my primary goal in writing this book. The ideas and suggestions here are just the tip of the iceberg, but if I have accomplished my goal, this information has compelled a patient, caregiver, or health-conscious individual to dig deeper, research more, boldly ask questions, and use every tool and resource available.

Above all, never give up, and never give in to illness. So many options have been unveiled, and the possibilities are seemingly endless to posture the body to heal. Now, boldly and with courage, take charge, pull out all the stops, turn every stone, and travel a new pathway!

Chapter 18

STEPS IN A NEW DIRECTION

T he healing process begins the moment necessary elements are realized and utilized. The miracle of miraculous recovery has been experienced by multitudes of people. Individuals vary, but the healing process is the same. There are so many ideas, practices, and modalities available for healing. Here is a review and the jump start on what I consider the fundamentals of recovery.

Enzymes: Incorporate a raw food into every meal, preferably a vegetable; choose berries if the raw food is fruit. At the end of this chapter, I have added a few of my favorite recipes that I feel have the highest nutritional impact and are a cinch to incorporate into a healthy diet regimen.

Alkalinity: Move away from an acidic body to an alkaline body. Support the body's natural 7.365 pH by adding minerals to the daily diet and minimizing sugar. Sugar is acid forming. Minerals are essential for the body to utilize vitamins, antioxidants, and other nutrients. Many minerals need other minerals present to be utilized properly. Minerals for humans must come from plant sources as humans can utilize minerals only from plant synthesis. This is why vegetables are the main focus of every diet. Eating vegetables in all the colors of the rainbow for the wonderful benefits they provide to our complex biochemical body is crucial. Squeeze a lemon or lime on the vegetables, and you have a wonderful base for alkaline-forming foods. Supplement your diet with quality, food-based multi-minerals if eating balanced is a struggle. Test urine with pH test strips along the way for quality control.

Hydration and salt: Drink at least three bottles of water a day with a pinch of Himalayan sea salt or Celtic sea salt to replenish the body's fluids and essential trace minerals at the same time. The water becomes alkaline with the salts. The sea salts are healthy and needed. Eliminate ordinary table salt completely. The water should not taste salty; it should be just a mild saline solution in harmony with the body's saline-like fluid. Drink this as part of your normal fluid intake; remember the standard measure of proper hydration is one-half of your body weight in ounces of water a day.

Sleep: Adding minerals, especially magnesium and calcium, to your before-bedtime routine provides the right combination at the right time for the body. Sleep is when the body heals, regenerates, and detoxifies. Taking a warm Epsom salt bath, having an herbal decaffeinated tea, listening to Zen-like music, cooling the room, getting very comfortable, and possibly adding melatonin, 5-HTP, or a sleep-essential supplement will support a prolonged period of deep sleep. This area of health varies drastically from individual to individual, and if the individual is on medication, especially for anxiety or depression, consulting a doctor before supplementation is imperative. Remember when supplementing with melatonin that it may cause vivid dreams or nightmares if the dosage is too low. Start low and work up. Eventually the body may start making enough melatonin naturally, and supplementing can be eliminated. Most important, don't give up until good, healthy, and consistent sleep is commonplace.

Stress: Supporting the body's delicate pH balance with food is important, but food alone can't reverse the effects of prolonged stressful thoughts. Stress and worry are large contributors of adrenal failure, fatigue, extreme weight gain or loss, sleeplessness, illness, and disease. When the body is stressed from mental or physical activity, it produces more cortisol, and this acid-forming hormone creates an inflammatory response. Eliminate stress. Making the sphere of people in your life smaller is a good start. Minimizing the time spent with stress-filled and chaos-causing individuals is good medicine and may be totally necessary to achieve pH balance. Remove clutter from the places where most of your time is spent. The car, kitchen, bathroom, family room, and office should be targeted first. Keep them organized and tidy, and eventually, if time allows, work on other areas. Accomplishing and maintaining order in these areas will bring about a sweet peace.

Elimination: Just like sleep, elimination varies immensely from individual to individual. Following common sense that what goes in must come out is the best approach here. Waste that stays in the body is incredibly damaging. Eliminating a bit after every meal with a formed stool is healthy. Anything short of that requires attention until success and consistency are experienced.

Go gluten free: Removing wheat is imperative to recovery. Removing this element, which is largely responsible for craving sugar and carbohydrates, from the diet is an ultimate factor in turning health around. Going gluten free aids in the reduction of inflammation and stopping the up and down cycles of craving in the body for starchy, sweet foods, which lead to fatigue and to needing caffeine for an energy boost. This is the perfect combo for acid reflux, bouts of deep fatigue, and potential adrenal, hormone, and blood-glucose-level dysfunction. The genetically modified gliadin protein added to wheat adds to the unhealthy cycle because it attaches to the opiate receptors in the brain and stimulates cravings.

Once the body is gluten and gliadin free, which comes with a wheat-free diet, the body's natural system of signaling what it needs when it needs it will work properly. The taste, smell, and popularity of healthier foods will become more intense and enjoyable, adding more to the list of benefits.

Go for the coconuts: Getting coconut-based nutrition incorporated into your every day will aid in getting more minerals, vitamins, and nutrients directly into your bloodstream. If the thought of anything coconut is lousy, use refined coconut oil in cooking and baking as it has no coconut flavor. If coconut is divine to you, go crazy on coconut products for overall better recovery. Forget the old dogma. Coconut is not a harmful, saturated fat as it was once considered. Coconut water hydrates the body faster, and coconut oil, milk, and shredded coconut aid in taking nutrition right into the blood and right into the cells.

The ABCs of alkaline healing are awareness, balance, and common sense. Eat simply. Live simply. Pause, slow down, breathe, smile, and dedicate this crucial time to slowing the aging process and recovering from illness. Live vibrantly as an example to others of total health transformation.

THREE RECIPES FOR
HEALTH TRANSFORMATION

SIMPLE.NATURAL.HEALING.RECIPE

Wellness Salad

One/Day Health Transformation

1 hard boiled egg or ½ cup plain Greek yogurt
1 oz. of Dark Chocolate (70% cacao or higher)
or cup of black regular coffee or both
2 oz. Strawberries, oranges, or blueberries
4 oz. Raspberries or carrots
1 oz. Apple
1 oz. Pineapple or orange
1 handful of baby greens or romaine lettuce
can sprinkle with Himalayan sea salt
option: 1 tsp. Bragg's Apple Cider vinegar for dressing
Put greens down and put all fruit on top - eat egg and chocolate along with the salad. For variety, the egg/yogurt can be replaced with meat, fish or nuts.

***This salad has shown to be very effective in health improvement in just 30 days, eaten once or twice per day.**

Health Benefits of Ingredients:

Eggs - A source of high quality protein, choline (good for liver health), vitamin B12, phosphorus and riboflavin.
Greek yogurt - Twice the protein, half the sodium and half the carbohydrates of regular yogurt. Natural probiotic for healthy gut.
Dark Chocolate 70% cacao - One of the best antioxidents in the world.
Black coffee - Reduces inflammation, beneficial antioxident, increases dopamine and enhances firing of neurons.
Strawberries - Vitamin C, folate, potassium, manganese & magnesium.
Oranges - Vitamin C, vitamin A, fiber, folate, vitamin B1, potassium, copper, pantothenic acid and calcium.
Blueberries - Vitamin C & manganese helps body process cholesterol.
Raspberries - Ellagic acid, vitamin C, quercetin and gallic acid.
Carrots - Vitamin A, vit. C, vit. K, vit. B8, potassium, iron, and folate.
Apple - Antioxidents, flavanoids, fiber linked to lower bad cholesterol.
Pineapple - Rich in many vitamins, minerals, enzymes and soluble fiber.
Greens & Romaine - Vit. K prevents hardening of arteries, many B vitamins, protein, omega-3 fatty acid and minerals.
Himalayan sea salt - Healthy utilizable salt and 84 trace minerals.
Bragg's Apple Cider vinegar - Potassium and balanced glucose levels.

Blood Sugar Stabilizer

1 16 oz. jar of almond butter
1/2 cup of melted coconut oil
1/4 cup coconut sugar
2 T. cinnamon
1/2 tsp. Himalayan sea salt

Mix well and store covered
*Optional 1/2 c. shredded coconut and/or 1/2 cup chopped
Pecans, walnuts or sunflower seeds
Serve on celery or carrot sticks

Health Benefits of Ingredients:

Almond butter - Alkaline source of protein, vitamin E and oxygen flow.
Coconut oil - Healthy saturated fat, raises good cholesterol (HDL), and lowers bad (LDL), stable oil that does not smoke at high temperatures and does not become rancid. It has antibacterial, anti-fungal and anti-microbial properties. Other oils must be broken down before they can be absorbed, coconut oil is easily digested, highly absorbable, does not need enzymes or bile for digestion. Good for gallbladder problems and diabetes. Coconut oil also increases immunity.
Coconut sugar - A low glycemic level natural sugar with a fiber called inulin which slows glucose absorption.
Cinnamon - Lowers blood sugar levels, lowers bad cholesterol (LDL), effective against yeast infections (Candida albicans fungus), stomach flu for it's antibacterial properties, reduces bloating, cancer prevention and fighter, eases pain of arthritis, natural food preservative, odor neutralizer, promotes alertness and cognitive memory, powerful antioxidant as well as a weight loss aid, good for blood circulation and boosts metabolism.
Himalayan sea salt - Healthy pH salt for digestion and absorption with 84 trace minerals, easily absorbed into the bloodstream with the presence of coconut oil and coconut sugar.
Nuts and seeds add protein and more minerals and nutrients to the mix.
Celery - Lowers stress hormones, reduces blood pressure, reduces bad cholesterol (LDL), good for bladder and kidney disorders, prevents urinary tract infections (UTI's). Good for asthma as anti-inflammatory.

SIMPLE.NATURAL.HEALING.RECIPE

Healthy Berry Coleslaw

1 bag of cabbage shredded or small head of cabbage chopped
2 shredded or chopped carrots
2 stalks of celery diced
1 container of strawberries cleaned and sliced (can use blueberries or both)
1 cup nuts (I use Pecans because I love them)
1 cup shredded coconut
1 single serving container of Greek yogurt (I use Greek coconut yogurt)
1/4 cup Rice Vinegar

- Mix yogurt and rice vinegar and set aside.
- Mix all other ingredients together in a nice big serving bowl.
- Mix yogurt/rice vinegar dressing through salad thoroughly and serve.

Health Benefits of Ingredients:

Cabbage - Cruciferous vegetable high in vitamin C, manganese, vitamin K, folate, fiber, potassium, sulphur, enzymes and antioxidants. Excellent anti-inflammatory and blood sugar regulator.

Carrots - Vitamin A, vitamin C, vitamin K, vitamin B8, potassium, iron, carotene, fiber and folate.

Celery - Low in calories, lowers stress hormones, reduces blood pressure, reduces bad cholesterol (LDL), good for bladder and kidney disorders, prevents urinary tract infections (UTI's), good for asthma, reduces cancer risk and degeneration of vision.

Strawberries - Vitamin C, folate, potassium, manganese and magnesium. Improves immune system, reduces signs of premature aging, and provides relief from gout, arthritis, high blood pressure. Strawberries also improve eye and brain function.

Pecans - Contains 19 vitamins, minerals and fiber. A rich antioxidant and heart healthy fat and is high in protein.

Coconut - Healthy fat and fiber with iron and zinc. Helps maintain healthy tissue and fights infections and disease.

Greek yogurt - Twice the protein, half the sodium, and fewer carbs than regular yogurt. Natural probiotic for healthy gut.

Rice Vinegar - Good weight control and limits sodium intake.

ABOUT THE AUTHOR

When author Donna LaBar shares her thirty years of study into nutritional healing, her eyes light up and her beauty defies her true age. A lifetime resident of the rural Pennsylvania town of Tunkhannock, LaBar is sought after for healing information on cancer, arthritis, weight loss, and more. She believes in the body's ability to heal when given the right nutrition, alkaline/acid balance, enzymes, environment, exercise, better sleep, and targeted stress reduction.

LaBar is a master of translating scientific healing health approaches into layman's terms. She receives calls for help every week from people who do not know where else to turn. Her gentle nutritional and healing guidance is recognized for its effectiveness, as shown in the stories she shares in *Simple. Natural. Healing.* She is self-taught in the field of medicinal properties of nutrition. Find out more about her life work at www.donnalabar.com.

A free eBook edition is available with the purchase of this book.

To claim your free eBook edition:

1. Download the Shelfie app.
2. Write your name in uppser case in the box.
3. Use the Shelfie app to submit a photo.
4. Download your eBook to any device.

Print & Digital Together Forever.

Snap a photo

Free eBook

Read anywhere

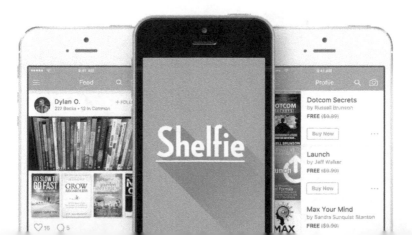

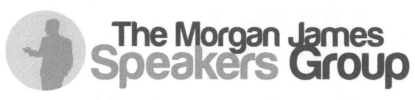

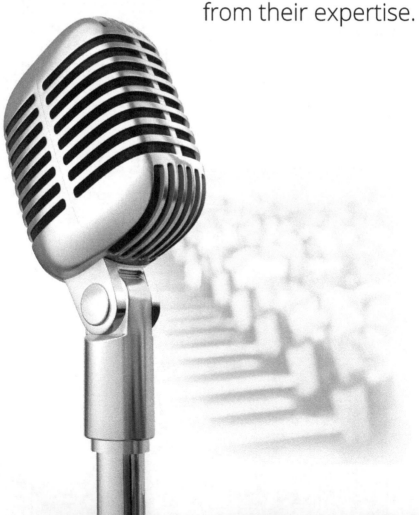

Morgan James makes all of our titles available
through the Library for All Charity Organization.

www.LibraryForAll.org

Printed in the USA
CPSIA information can be obtained
at www.ICGtesting.com
JSHW082352140824
68134JS00020B/2028